The
Hypothyroid
Sourcebook

Other books by M. Sara Rosenthal

The Thyroid Sourcebook (4th ed., 2000)

The Gynecological Sourcebook (3d ed., 1999)

The Pregnancy Sourcebook (3d ed., 1999)

The Fertility Sourcebook (3d ed., 1999)

The Breastfeeding Sourcebook (3d ed., 1999)

The Breast Sourcebook (2d ed., 1999)

The Gastrointestinal Sourcebook (1997; 1998)

The Type 2 Diabetic Woman (U.S. only; 1999)

The Thyroid Sourcebook for Women (1999)

Women and Depression (2000)

Women of the '60s Turning 50 (2000)

Women and Passion (2000)

Managing PMS Naturally (2001)

The Canadian Type 2 Diabetes Sourcebook (Canada only; 2001)

50 Ways Series

50 Ways to Prevent Colon Cancer (2000)

50 Ways Women Can Prevent Heart Disease (2000)

50 Ways to Manage Ulcer, Heartburn and Reflux (2001)

50 Ways to Manage Type 2 Diabetes (U.S. only; 2001)

50 Ways to Prevent and Manage Stress (2001)

50 Ways to Fight Depression Without Drugs (2002)

SarahealthGuides™ These are M. Sara Rosenthal's own line of health books dedicated to rare, controversial, or stigmatizing health topics you won't find in regular bookstores. SarahealthGuides™ are available only at online bookstores such as amazon.com. Visit sarahealth.com for upcoming titles.

Stopping Cancer at the Source (2001)

Women and Unwanted Hair (2001)

The
Hypothyroid
Sourcebook

M. SARA ROSENTHAL, M.S.

author of *The Thyroid Sourcebook for Women* and *The Thyroid Sourcebook*

Contemporary Books

Chicago New York San Francisco Lisbon London Madrid Mexico City
Milan New Delhi San Juan Seoul Singapore Sydney Toronto

Library of Congress Cataloging-in-Publication Data

Rosenthal, M. Sara.
    The hypothyroid sourcebook / M. Sara Rosenthal.
        p.   cm.
    Includes bibliographical references and index.
    ISBN 0-7373-0595-9
    1. Hypothyroidism—Popular works.   I. Title.

    RC657.R674   2002
    616.4'44—dc21   2001053692

Contemporary Books &

A Division of The McGraw-Hill Companies

1 2 3 4 5 6 7 8 9 10   DOC/DOC   1 10 9 8 7 6 5 4 3 2

ISBN 0-7373-0595-9

This book was set in Sabon by Rattray Design
Printed and bound by R. R. Donnelley—Crawfordsville

Cover design by Jeanette Wojtyla

McGraw-Hill books are available at special quantity discounts to use as premiums and sales promotions, or for use in corporate training programs. For more information, please write to the Director of Special Sales, Professional Publishing, McGraw-Hill, Two Penn Plaza, New York, NY 10121-2298. Or contact your local bookstore.

Important Notice: The purpose of this book is to educate. It is sold with the understanding that the author and publisher shall have neither liability nor responsibility for any injury caused or alleged to be caused directly or indirectly by the information contained in this book. While every effort has been made to ensure its accuracy, the book's contents should not be construed as medical advice. Each person's health needs are unique. To obtain recommendations appropriate to your particular situation, please consult a qualified health care provider. Any herbal information in this book is provided for education purposes only and is not meant to be used without consulting a qualified health practitioner who is trained in herbal medicine.

This book is printed on acid-free paper.

Contents

Acknowledgments

I WISH TO thank the following people (listed alphabetically), whose expertise and dedication as medical advisors on previous works helped to lay so much of the groundwork for this book:

Gillian Arsenault, M.D., C.C.F.P., I.B.L.C., F.R.C.P.
Pamela Craig, M.D., F.A.C.S., Ph.D.
Susan George, M.D., F.R.C.P., F.A.C.P.
Masood Khathamee, M.D., F.A.C.O.G.
Gary May, M.D., F.R.C.P.
James McSherry, M.B., Ch.B., F.C.F.P., F.R.C.G.P., F.A.A.F.P., F.A.B.M.P.
Debra Lander, M.D., F.R.C.P.
Matthew Lazar, M.D., F.R.C.P., F.A.C.P.
Suzanne Pratt, M.D., F.A.C.O.G.
Irving B. Rosen, M.D., F.R.C.S., F.A.C.S.
Wm. Warren Rudd, M.D., F.R.C.S., F.A.C.S.
Robert Volpe, M.D., F.R.C.P., F.A.C.P.

I'd also like to thank Kelly Hale, Executive Director/Founder, American Foundation of Thyroid Patients, for her continuous support.

Larissa Kostoff, Editorial Consultant on this book, worked very hard to make this book come to fruition.

And finally, I continue to appreciate the support that comes from my friends and family members.

Introduction

As a THYROID cancer survivor (I was diagnosed at age twenty in 1983), I live without a thyroid gland and have battled with long bouts of hypothyroidism. When I wrote the first comprehensive book on thyroid disease for the consumer, *The Thyroid Sourcebook* (now in its fourth edition), it was 1993. At that time, there were no books on thyroid disease written by someone who actually *had* the disease. The doctor-authored books were either too sparse or too technical for the average reader and unavailable in mainstream bookstores. *The Thyroid Sourcebook* was designed as a one-stop resource on all forms of thyroid disease and cancer—in nontechnical language. And it has benefited more people than I ever imagined. In 1999, I was able to add to the thyroid bookshelf *The Thyroid Sourcebook for Women*, a book I strongly believed was needed, as thyroid disease is roughly ten times more common in women.

In 2000, another significant thyroid book hit the shelves: *Living Well with Hypothyroidism* by Mary Shomon, thyroid sufferer (and kindred spirit) who is a strong grassroots patient advocate for thyroid disease on the Internet. Mary's book flew off the shelves and quickly became a bestseller. Clearly, providing thyroid information from a patient's perspective is appreciated!

The *Hypothyroid Sourcebook* is meant as a complement to your growing thyroid library. I have provided unique information you will not read elsewhere, and where necessary, I refer you to *The Thyroid Sourcebook* or *The Thyroid Sourcebook for Women*. I have created The Hypothyroid Diet (Chapter 4), The Hypothyroid Active Living Program (Chapter 5), and The Hypothyroid Herbal and Wellness Program (Chapter 6) to help you manage your hypothyroidism. This is to add to the good information on this disorder that for many years was ignored by health publishers. I took cues from numerous readers' letters and E-mails asking for a more proactive "plan" for dealing with hypothyroidism.

In my own journey with health writing and patient advocacy, I became interested in the field of health promotion and bioethics. In 2000, I launched my own health promotion Web site, www.sara health.com, which soon will be publishing books devoted to rare, stigmatizing, or controversial health conditions (look for books on thyroid cancer, Graves' disease, and thyroid eye disease). I also became a bioethicist, which has allowed me to contribute to patients' rights and advocate for thyroid disease sufferers in ways I never dreamed possible.

Anyone dealing with thyroid disease may also be faced with a myriad of other health concerns. Be aware that you are not just entitled to information, but you are legally owed information. Being informed about medical tests and procedures is known as "informed consent," a guiding principle for medical practitioners and researchers. It means that to make an informed decision there must be full disclosure of all risks and benefits; you must completely understand what's being explained; you must be fully competent; and you must feel free to say "yes" or "no" according to your own wishes, values, and "gut feeling" without any coercion or coaxing.

Most medical ethicists agree that informed consent is an oxymoron, like "jumbo shrimp"; the two ideas are incompatible. Because to be truly informed when it comes to medical procedures (thyroid or otherwise), it's often not enough to know "what time it is"; you need to know how to build a watch. The problem with "informed consent" is that unless *you* are a doctor, how informed can you be?

Before you consent to any medical test, procedure, or treatment, your doctor should disclose the following:

- a description of the test, procedure, or treatment and its expected effects (for example, duration of hospital stay, expected time to recovery, restrictions on daily activities, scars)
- information about relevant alternative options and their expected benefits and relevant risks
- explanation of the consequences of declining or delaying treatment

Your doctor should also be giving you an opportunity to ask questions—and should be available to answer them.

Here are all the questions you must ask yourself:

1. Do *you* understand the information relevant to your decision? Do you appreciate the reasonably foreseeable consequences of your decision or *lack* of decision? This is what is known as your *capacity* to consent to procedures.
2. Do you understand what's being disclosed? Can you make your decision based on this information?
3. Are you being allowed to make your decision free of any undue influences? (For example, are you in pain? Is information being distorted or omitted? Are you being sedated?) This is what is known as *voluntariness*; involuntary consent means, of course, that you haven't consented to a procedure.

If you answer "no" to any of these questions, you are probably not being given adequate information, or you are in no shape to make a decision about your health. But as a thyroid patient today, you have the benefit of being able to find many good books and other sources for information on this disease. Take advantage of *all* the material available—and educate yourself. Let *The Hypothyroid Sourcebook* be one of your guiding lights to good health.

The
Hypothyroid
Sourcebook

1

Why Am I Hypothyroid?

HYPOTHYROID MEANS THAT your thyroid gland is underactive and is not making enough thyroid hormone for your body's requirements. If you've been diagnosed with a thyroid disorder, you will probably experience hypothyroidism at some point. There are two categories of people who become hypothyroid. The first category is what I call "side-effect hypothyroidism." Anyone who is treated for hyperthyroidism (an overactive thyroid gland) will become hypothyroid if the thyroid gland is destroyed with radioactive iodine. Anyone treated for thyroid cancer will also become hypothyroid if the thyroid gland is removed. For more information on hyperthyroidism, thyroid cancer, or nodules on the thyroid, refer to my books *The Thyroid Sourcebook, 4th edition,* or *The Thyroid Sourcebook for Women.*

Roughly 25 to 50 percent of all people who have received external radiation therapy to the head and neck area for cancers such as Hodgkin's disease tend to develop hypothyroidism within five years after their treatment. It's recommended that this group have an annual thyroid stimulating hormone (TSH) test. For more on TSH testing, see later in this chapter. Sometimes hypothyroidism occurs because of a pituitary gland disorder, which may interfere with the production of thyrotropin-releasing hormone (TRH). This is pretty rare, however. Tumors or cysts on the pituitary gland can also interfere with thyroid hormone production.

The second category of hypothyroidism is what I call "primary hypothyroidism." By this, I refer to people who develop hypothyroidism as a primary condition, unrelated to any medical treatments they have had for other thyroid disorders. This group includes people who develop thyroiditis (inflammation of the thyroid gland) from Hashimoto's disease (see further on), babies born without a thyroid gland, or people who stop making as much thyroid hormone as they used to due to aging. I will cover all conditions resulting in primary hypothyroidism further on, but first let's review what the thyroid gland is!

What's a Thyroid?

The thyroid was named in the 1600s, and is Greek for "shield" because of its butterfly shape. Your thyroid gland is located in the lower part of your neck, in front of your windpipe (see Figure 1.1), and it produces two thyroid hormones—thyroxine, known as T4 (four iodine atoms), and triiodothyronine, known as T3 (three iodine atoms). Although there are two hormones, thyroid hormone is referred to in the singular (the word *hormone* is Greek for "stimulator"). Thyroid hormone is secreted into the circulation and becomes widely distributed throughout the body. It is one of the basic regulators of the functions of every cell and every tissue within the body, and a steady supply is crucial for good health (see Figure 1.2). In essence, your thyroid affects you from head to toe—including your skin and hair!

If you were to break down exactly how much T4 and T3 is secreted by your thyroid, you'd find that 90 percent of the thyroid output is T4, and only 10 percent is T3. Although these hormones have the same effect in your body, T3 is four times as powerful as T4 and works *eight times* as fast. It's akin to juice in a bottle and frozen concentrate. T4 can also "turn into" T3 by shedding an iodine atom if your body quickly requires some thyroid hormone.

Iodine

Your thyroid gland extracts iodine from various foods, including certain vegetables, shellfish, milk products (cow udders are washed with large

Figure 1.1 *Where Your Thyroid Lives*

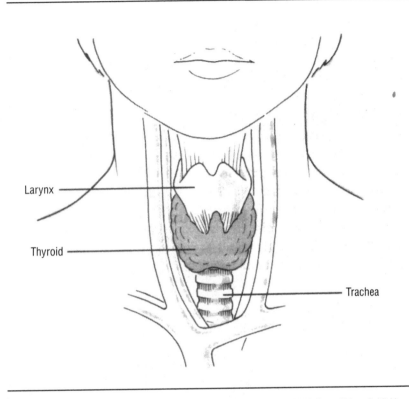

Larynx

Thyroid

Trachea

amounts of iodine, which winds up in your milk), and *anything* with iodized salt. Normally, we take in sufficient iodine through our diet.

Our thyroids are very sensitive to iodine. When the thyroid gland is not able to obtain sufficient quantities of iodine, your thyroid can enlarge and you develop what is called a goiter. A goiter could develop if your thyroid gland absorbs too much iodine, and produces either too little or too much thyroid hormone. Although it seems odd that too much or too little iodine can produce the same results, the reason the goiter develops is different in each case. Usually, where too little iodine is present a goiter is caused by an increased activity of thyroid gland cells, while too much iodine can cause the thyroid gland to enlarge.

Figure 1.2 The Thyroid Affects the Body from Head to Toe

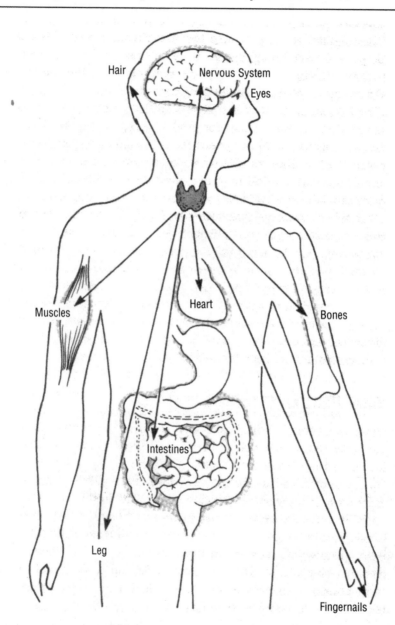

Goiter Belts and Iodine Deficiency

A goiter belt is not a fashion accessory. It refers to geographical regions that typically supply insufficient iodine. The Great Lakes region, for example, was considered a goiter belt. The term originated because inhabitants of these regions would often develop goiters from a lack of iodine. Goiter belts are far from salt water. In regions close to salt water, iodine gets into the soil and the water supplies from wind and the rain off salty seas, and it also gets into the plants. It then travels into the milk and meat that we eat.

The introduction of iodized salt in our diet has virtually eliminated goiters from iodine deficiencies in North America. But the problem of iodine deficiency is far from solved in other parts of the world. In fact, over one billion people are at risk for iodine deficiency–related thyroid disease. Three hundred million people in Asia alone suffer from goiters, while twenty million people suffer from brain damage due to iodine deficiency in pregnancy and infancy. This is very disturbing, since these problems can be completely prevented by the simple addition of iodized salt or iodized oil (proposed in some regions) to the diet. Goiters from iodine deficiency are regularly found in Asia, Africa, and South America, especially in mountainous regions such as the Himalayas and the Andes.

The first International Goiter Congress was held in 1929 in Berne after Switzerland and the United States introduced iodized salt. Many countries soon followed and iodine deficiency disappeared in most parts of the world. Not much happened to eliminate iodine deficiency in underdeveloped nations until 1985, when thyroid specialists established the International Council for Control of Iodine Deficiency Disorders (ICCIDD), a group of about four hundred members from seventy different countries.

In North America, about one in four thousand newborns is born with hypothyroidism; in iodine-deficient areas, 10 percent of all newborns are hypothyroid. Worse, up to 70 percent of the iodine-deficient populations are severely hypothyroid. Iodine deficiency is now recognized as the most common cause of preventable mental defects. ICCIDD works with the World Health Organization and UNICEF to develop national programs in Africa, Asia, Latin America, and Europe whose goal is elimination of iodine deficiency in the near future. Most recently, the salt industry has joined in the fight.

A current project under way is the European ThyroMobil Campaign, which visits areas that are plagued with iodine deficiency. The company that runs the van has developed a urine test for iodine deficiency that delivers results in ten minutes.

The Role of Calcitonin

Your thyroid gland rents space to nonthyroid cells called C cells, which make the hormone calcitonin. This hormone helps to regulate calcium, hence helping to prevent osteoporosis. It is also used to treat Paget's disease, a bone disease that affects mostly men. But to your *bones*, calcitonin is kind of like a tonsil; it serves a useful purpose, but when the hormone is not manufactured due to the absence of a thyroid gland (if it's removed or ablated by radioactive iodine), you won't really notice any effects, just as you don't "miss" your tonsils. Calcium levels are really controlled by the parathyroid glands (discussed further on), and is much more dependent on the hormone estrogen, which helps with calcium absorption, diet, and exercise, and builds bone mass.

Calcitonin is only important when discussing the thyroid if you're discussing screening for a rare type of thyroid cancer called medullary thyroid cancer (see *The Thyroid Sourcebook, 4th edition*).

The Role of Thyroglobulin

Although the name sounds like a Halloween candy, thyroglobulin is a specific protein made only by your thyroid cells, used mostly by the thyroid gland itself to make thyroid hormone. Like calcitonin, this substance isn't all that important to your body once your thyroid is gone; you won't miss it. The only role thyroglobulin plays after your thyroid problem is treated is in screening for thyroid cancer *recurrence*. (See *The Thyroid Sourcebook, 4th edition.*) For hypothyroid or hyperthyroid patients, however, screening for thyroglobulin is useless.

The Pituitary Gland

Your thyroid is under a lot of pressure to meet exact demand for a product it monopolizes. That's where your pituitary gland comes in to play. Like a government, it controls and regulates all bodily functions and secretions. The pituitary gland, often referred to as the master gland, is situated at the base of the skull and is, without question, the most influential gland in your body. Your thyroid gland directly reports to it.

The pituitary gland regularly monitors T4 and T3 stock in your body's blood levels. When stock is low, it sends a message to your thyroid gland—in the form of a stimulating hormone called TSH (thyroid-stimulating hormone)—and orders it to produce more. The pituitary gland will only secrete increased amounts of TSH when T4 and/or T3 levels are low.

The Causes of Primary Hypothyroidism

Primary hypothyroidism is most often caused by an autoimmune disorder known as Hashimoto's disease, which causes inflammation of the thyroid gland. Here, we will look closely at all the conditions causing primary hypothyroidism, but we will not cover "side-effect" hypothyroidism—hypothyroidism caused by medical treatments for other thyroid conditions. These are covered in *The Thyroid Sourcebook, 4th edition.*

Hashimoto's Disease

Also known as Hashimoto's thyroiditis or "chronic lymphocytic thyroiditis" (because of the involvement of self-attacking lymphocytes), this disease is named after Hakaru Hashimoto, the Japanese physician who first described the condition in 1912.

Hashimoto's disease is caused by abnormal blood antibodies and white blood cells attacking and damaging thyroid cells. Eventually, the constant attack destroys many of the thyroid cells. The absence of sufficient thyroid cells causes hypothyroidism. In most cases, a goiter develops because of the inflammation, but sometimes the thyroid gland can actually shrink.

If you develop Hashimoto's disease, you probably won't notice any symptoms at all. Sometimes there's a mild pressure in the thyroid gland and sometimes fatigue can set in, but unless you're on the lookout for a thyroid disease, Hashimoto's disease can go undetected for years. Only when the thyroid cells are damaged to the point that the thyroid gland functions inadequately will you begin to experience the symptoms of hypothyroidism, described further on.

In some rare instances, thyroid eye disease can set in as well (see *The Thyroid Sourcebook, 4th edition*). The antibodies produced in Hashimoto's disease most likely aggravate the proteins in the eye muscle. Treating eye problems associated with Hashimoto's disease involves treating the initial hypothyroidism first.

Rarer still, some people with Hashimoto's disease experience hyperthyroidism *as well as* hypothyroidism. This hyper/hypo "combo platter" happens because sometimes there are two forces of antibodies at work: those that attack and destroy the thyroid cells, and those that stimulate the gland to overproduce thyroxine—exactly like the antibodies involved with Graves' disease. This condition is coined "Hashitoxicosis." Anyone suffering from this somewhat paradoxical condition would *first* experience all the symptoms of hyperthyroidism. Usually, after a few months, the antibodies attacking the thyroid cells overpower the Graves'-like antibodies, and the hyperthyroidism cures itself. Then, as Hashimoto's disease progresses, you'd eventually wind up hypothyroid unless replacement hormone was prescribed.

Diagnosis and Treatment of Hashimoto's Disease

The signs of Hashimoto's disease are not at all obvious. In the early stage, a goiter can develop as a result of inflammation in the thyroid gland. The goiter is usually firm, but in rare cases it can actually be tender. The tenderness of the goiter can suggest Hashimoto's, but usually Hashimoto's disease is suspected because of a sudden hypothyroidism, or because of the age of a hypothyroid patient.

Hashimoto's disease is easily diagnosed through a blood test that detects high levels of antibodies in the blood. Another method of confirming a diagnosis of Hashimoto's disease is a needle biopsy. Here, a needle is inserted into the thyroid gland to remove some of its cells. The cells are smeared onto a glass slide; in the case of Hashimoto's disease, you would see abnormal white blood cells.

The treatment is simple: thyroid replacement hormone is prescribed (see Chapter 3) as soon as the diagnosis is made—even if there are no symptoms. There are three reasons why this is done. First, the synthetic hormone suppresses production of thyroid-stimulating hormone (TSH) by the pituitary gland, which, in turn, shrinks any goiter that may have developed, or is about to develop. Second, because Hashimoto's disease often progresses to the point where hypothyroidism sets in, the synthetic hormone nips the hypothyroidism in the bud and prevents the Hashimoto's patient from suffering the unpleasant symptoms of hypothyroidism. Finally, for some reason, synthetic thyroid hormone seems to interfere with the blood antibodies that are attacking the thyroid gland.

If you've developed a goiter as a result of Hashimoto's disease, it will usually persist until thyroid hormone is prescribed. Occasionally the goiter shrinks on its own. On the average, it takes anywhere from six to eighteen months for a goiter to shrink, and when it does you'll most certainly be hypothyroid. Most often, a shrunken thyroid gland is small from the beginning. (Remember, a goiter is simply an enlarged thyroid gland, so when the thyroid gland shrivels up, it no longer functions.) In rare instances, goiters can persist for years—despite synthetic thyroid hormone.

More on Autoimmune Disorders

The word *autoimmune* means "self-attacking." But before you can really grasp what this means, it's important to understand how your body normally fights off infection or disease.

Whenever an invading virus or cell is detected, your body produces specific "armies" called antibodies, which attack foreign intruders known as antigens. Antibodies are made from one type of white blood cell (called lymphocytes) and each antibody is designed for a specific virus, the way a key is designed for a specific lock. The antibody acts as the key, while the antigen, or "intruder," is the lock. For example, if you had contracted the chicken pox as a child, you couldn't contract it again; your body is armed with the antibody that kills the chicken pox virus. But the specific chicken pox antibody is useless against all other viruses, such as the mumps or measles.

Often, our doctors give us vaccines to prevent the development of a particular virus; polio, for example. Vaccines work like this: The serum contains a small amount of a particular virus in a deadened, noncontagious form. Essentially, a vaccine shows your body a picture of the virus—the way the police post the face of a "Wanted" fugitive. The vaccine serum stimulates your system to produce a specific antibody to combat against the "Wanted" virus. Later, if you catch the virus, your body destroys it before it can do any damage. That's why you don't need to get chicken pox to be protected from it; you can be vaccinated against it instead. However, creating a vaccine is a painstaking, complicated process, and it can take years for scientists to develop vaccines to specific viruses. Polio struck at epidemic proportions throughout the 1940s and 1950s until a vaccine was discovered.

With an autoimmune disorder, your body loses the ability to distinguish foreign tissue from normal tissue. It confuses the two, and perceives healthy organs as invading viruses. Your body then winds up attacking its own organs. Some doctors describe it as a sort of allergy, where your body is in fact allergic to itself. So in the same way that the body develops specific antibodies to fight specific infections, here the body develops specific antibodies to attack specific organs. These are also known as autoantibodies. Many kinds of illnesses are in fact autoimmune disorders; Hashimoto's disease is one of them.

Neonatal and Congenital Hypothyroidism

Roughly one in four thousand babies is born with either neonatal or congenital hypothyroidism, and they are different from one another. In the first case, the baby is born without a thyroid gland. In the second case, the baby is born with what appears to be a normal thyroid gland, but develops symptoms of hypothyroidism after its first twenty-eight days of life. This is known as *congenital hypothyroidism*, which is treated no differently from neonatal hypothyroidism. In this case, while the condition was *present* at birth, the symptoms didn't *manifest* until later. Congenital hypothyroidism is just as serious as neonatal hypothyroidism, and may not be obvious until brain damage has already set in.

Neonatal and congenital hypothyroidism are very serious conditions, because they can lead to severe brain damage and developmental impairment. They can occur from an iodine deficiency in the mother's diet. This is common in more remote or mountainous areas of the world where iodine is not readily available. In fact, iodine deficiency is the most common cause of mental retardation in underdeveloped countries. Fortunately, this is not a problem in North America, where all our salt is iodized. (And low-salt diets still contain enough iodine for our needs.) Furthermore, since neonatal screening for hypothyroidism in newborns was introduced in the mid-1970s through the "heelpad" test, we can now prevent congenital hypothyroidism.

Postpartum Thyroiditis

Postpartum thyroiditis means "inflammation of the thyroid gland after delivery" and is often the culprit behind the so-called "postpartum blues." It usually lasts six to nine months before it resolves on its own.

Postpartum thyroiditis is a general label referring to silent thyroiditis occurring after delivery. This is usually a short-lived, Hashimoto's-type of thyroiditis, causing mild hypothyroidism. Until quite recently, the mild hypothyroid symptoms were simply attributed to the symptoms of postpartum depression, thought to be caused by the dramatic hormonal changes women experience after pregnancy. But recent studies indicate that as many as 18 percent of all pregnant women experience transient (short-lived) thyroid problems, and subsequent mild forms of hyperthyroidism or hypothyroidism. This statistic does not account for the many women who develop thyroid disease either during or after pregnancy. Today, it should be standard practice for all pregnant women in North America to have their thyroid glands tested after delivery. For more information, see *The Thyroid Sourcebook for Women*.

Other Forms of Thyroiditis

Although the most common form of thyroiditis is Hashimoto's disease, other kinds can occur and cause either hypo- or hyperthyroidism. Depending on what kind of thyroiditis you have, a goiter and symptoms of hyperthyroidism or hypothyroidism can develop. Other forms of thyroiditis include:

- *Subacute Viral Thyroiditis* (also known as *de Quervain's thyroiditis*). It's suspected that subacute ("not-so-severe") viral thyroiditis is probably caused by one or more viruses. Although there is no final proof that this condition is viral in origin, several possible viruses have been implicated that are similar to the measles or mumps virus, and certain common cold viruses. The condition ranges from extremely mild to severe and usually runs its course the way a normal flu virus does. When the gland gets inflamed, thyroid hormones leak out of the thyroid gland, the way pus oozes out of a blister. Then your system has too much thyroid hormone and you experience the classic hyperthyroid symptoms outlined earlier. (See also Table 2.1 on pg. 39.) Sometimes damage to the thyroid gland can result in permanent hypothyroidism, which means that you will need to be on thyroid hormone replacement for life.

- *Silent Thyroiditis.* This silent form of thyroiditis is so named because it's tricky to diagnose. Silent thyroiditis runs a painless course but otherwise is similar to subacute viral thyroiditis. With this version, there are no symptoms or outward signs of inflammation, but mild hyperthyroidism still occurs—for the same leakage reasons. Usually silent thyroiditis sufferers are women, commonly in the postpartum period as discussed earlier. This is also sometimes referred to as *spontaneously resolving hyperthyroidism.*

Borderline Hypothyroidism

The medical term for this is subclinical hypothyroidism. It refers to hypothyroidism that hasn't progressed very far, which means you have no symptoms yet. On a blood test, your T4 (thyroid hormone) readings would be very close to normal, but your thyroid-stimulating hormone (TSH) readings would be high. Right now, there is much discussion in clinical circles about doing routine TSH testing in certain groups of people for subclinical hypothyroidism. This would include anyone with a family history of thyroid disease, women over forty, women after childbirth, and anyone over the age of sixty. Because the TSH test is so simple to do, and can be added to any blood lab package, this is an opportunity to "catch" hypothyroidism before symptoms develop, and prevent it, along with all the symptoms discussed below. When you examine the symptoms of hypothyroidism, fatigue and depression in particular can lead to some real problems with misdiagnosis—in both directions. Depression can mask hypothyroidism and vice versa. Chronic fatigue syndrome may also mask hypothyroidism and vice versa. For this reason, I've devoted Chapter 2 to ruling out other causes for hypothyroid symptoms.

Feeling Under Par: Hypo Symptoms

When you're hypothyroid, everything slows down—including your body temperature. Feeling cold all the time is one of the more classic hypothyroid symptoms. When your body slows down, there are equal but opposite symptoms to the hyperthyroid scenario. These symptoms are listed here alphabetically so you can easily find the information you need. The symptoms will disappear once the thyroid problem is treated.

Cardiovascular Changes

Hypothyroid people will have an unusually slow pulse (fifty to seventy beats per minute), and either low or high blood pressure.

More severe or prolonged hypothyroidism could raise your cholesterol levels as well, which can aggravate coronary arteries. In a severe hypothyroid picture, the heart muscle fibers may weaken, which can lead to heart failure. This scenario is rare, however; one would have to suffer from severe and obvious hypothyroid symptoms long before the heart would be at risk.

If you're past menopause, this may aggravate your risk for heart disease, since estrogen loss can lead to heart disease in women. For example, it's not unusual if you're hypothyroid to notice chest pain (which may be confused with angina), or shortness of breath when you exert yourself, and you may notice some calf pain as well, which is caused by hardening of the arteries in the leg. Fluid may also collect, causing swollen legs and feet.

Cold Intolerance

You may not be able to find a comfortable temperature, and may often wonder "why it's always so *freezing* in here?!" Hypothyroid people carry sweaters with them all the time to compensate for a continuous sensitivity to cold. You'll feel much more comfortable in hot, muggy weather, and you may not perspire at all in the heat. This is because your entire metabolic rate has slowed down as your body conserves heat by diverting blood away from your skin.

Depression and Psychiatric Misdiagnosis

Hypothyroidism is linked to psychiatric depression more frequently than hyperthyroidism. The physical symptoms associated with major depression (discussed in relation to hyperthyroidism) may signal a psychiatric misdiagnosis. Sometimes psychiatrists find that hypothyroid patients exhibit behaviors linked to psychosis, such as paranoia or aural and visual hallucinations (hearing voices, seeing things that aren't there). Interestingly, roughly 15 percent of all patients suffering from depression are found to be hypothyroid.

Digestive Changes and Weight Gain

Because your system is slowed down, you'll suffer from constipation, hardening of stools, bloating (which may cause bad breath), poor appetite, and heartburn. The heartburn results because your food is not moving through the stomach as quickly, so acid and reflux (where semidigested food comes up the esophagus) may occur.

Because the lack of thyroid hormone slows your metabolism, you might gain weight. But often, because your appetite may decrease radically, your weight stays the same. Hypothyroid patients can experience some or all of these symptoms, or, if hypothyroidism is suspected early enough, patients may not be conscious of any symptoms until their doctor specifically asks them if they've noticed a particular change in metabolism or energy. You'll need to adjust your eating habits to compensate (discussed in Chapter 4). The typical scenario is to gain ten pounds or so during a period of about a year, even though you may not be eating as much. Some of the weight gain, however, may be due to bloating from constipation.

Dizziness

Slow circulation and low blood pressure can lead to dizziness and even to fainting.

Enlarged Thyroid Gland

Your thyroid gland often enlarges because it's inflamed—especially if you have Hashimoto's disease (see earlier discussion). But sometimes the destruction of the thyroid tissue can actually cause the thyroid gland to shrink.

Fatigue and Sleepiness

The most classic symptom is a distinct, lethargic tiredness or sluggishness, causing you to feel unnaturally sleepy. I refer to my own hypothyroid symptoms as "ass draggy," where you want to sleep all the time, even though you slept well over twelve hours the night before. Your doctor may also notice very slow reflexes. Researchers now know that when you're hypothyroid, you are unable to reach the deepest "stage 4" level of sleep, which is the most restful kind. This is why you remain tired, sleepy, and unrefreshed.

Fingernails

Fingernails become brittle and develop lines and grooves to the point where nail polish becomes impossible.

Hair Changes

When you're hypothyroid, your hair may become thinner, dry, and brittle, causing you to need lots of hair conditioner. Hair loss may also occur to the point where balding sets in. You will also lose body hair, such as eyebrows, leg and arm hair, as well as pubic hair.

Hearing Problems

Ringing or whistling in the ear (called tinnitus) affects roughly two-thirds of the hypothyroid population, while about one-third may actually suffer hearing loss. This is apparently due to a shortage of thyroid hormone in the nerves.

High Cholesterol

Hypothyroid people can easily develop high cholesterol, which can lead to a host of problems, including heart disease. This should be controlled through diet until your thyroid problem comes under control. It's generally recommended to anyone with high cholesterol to be tested for hypothyroidism.

Hives

This tends to occur with thyroid patients who have either hyper- or hypothyroidism. Hives are harmless, red, itchy welts on the skin. Antihistamines usually take care of the problem.

Menstrual Cycle Changes

Menstrual periods become much heavier and more frequent than usual, and sometimes ovaries can stop producing an egg each month. This can make conception difficult, if you're trying to have a child. For more details, see *The Thyroid Sourcebook for Women*.

Muscles

Common complaints from hypothyroid people are muscular aches and cramps (which may contribute to crampier periods in women). Many people believe they are experiencing arthritic symptoms. The aching can be severe enough to wake you up at night, but this condition completely clears up once hypothyroidism is treated. Muscle coordination is also a problem, where you feel "clutzy" all the time and find it hard to carry out simple motor tasks.

Numbness

This is combined with the sensation of pins and needles, as well as a tendency to develop *carpal tunnel syndrome*, characterized by tingling and numbness in the hands. It's caused in this case by compression on nerves in the wrist, due to water retention and bloating. This condition also plagues pregnant women, who suffer from water retention. Carpal tunnel syndrome is a repetitive strain injury and can be aggravated by typing, for example. This condition should go away once your hypothyroidism is treated.

Poor Memory and Concentration

Hypothyroidism causes a "spacey" feeling, where you may find it difficult to remember things, or to concentrate on a task. This is especially scary for seniors, who may feel as though dementia is setting in. In fact, one of the most common causes of so-called "senility" can be undiagnosed hypothyroidism. So before you shout "Alzheimer's," get a thyroid function test for the loved one you suspect is "losing it."

Skin Changes

Skin may feel dry and coarse to the point where it flakes like powder when you scratch it. Cracked skin will also become the norm on your elbows and kneecaps. Your skin will sport a yellowish hue as hypothyroidism worsens. The yellow comes from a buildup of carotene, a substance in our diet that normally gets converted into vitamin A, a process that slows down due to hypothyroidism. Because your body is conserving heat, and diverting blood away from your skin, you'll look pale and washed out.

Other symptoms more obvious to a physician would be the presence of a condition known as myxedema, the thickening of the skin and underlying tissues. Myxedema is characterized by a puffiness around the eyes and face, and can even involve the tongue, which also enlarges.

Stunted Growth in Children

The classic scenario is wondering why your twelve-year-old son still looks like he's only nine. So you take him to the doctor, and find out that his thyroid petered out, and he's stopped growing! This completely reverses once treatment with thyroid hormone begins.

Voice Changes

If your thyroid is enlarged, it may affect your vocal cords, causing your voice to sound hoarse or husky.

Testing Your Thyroid Function

Testing for hypothyroidism is done through a simple blood test called the TSH test. Whether you live in the United States or Canada, there is now a home TSH testing kit available through a company called Biosafe Laboratories, Inc. The test is done through a simple prick of a finger, similar to blood sugar testing. A recent national survey revealeed that almost 60 percent of Americans have never been tested for a thyroid condition. For more information on home TSH test kits, contact the Biosafe Web site http://www.ebiosafe.com, or call 1-888-700-TEST (8378). A normal TSH reading ranges from 0.5 to 5. A reading greater than 5 suggests that you're hypothyroid, while a reading less than 0.5 suggests that you're hyperthyroid (meaning that your gland is overactive). The word "normal" is highly subjective in medicine. You can fall outside the TSH range (either lower or higher) and feel hypothyroid and told you're not. Or, you may be told you're hypothyroid but feel just fine. Much of what we know about general health is that which is normal for a white male's body, because those who participated in clinical trials looking at diseases, treatments, drug studies, interactions, and so on used to be white males. Keep that in mind when you go for any medical test and are told you are "normal" when you do not feel that you're functioning normally for you. There are other tests that can confirm or help shed light on whether you are hypothyroid. They include tests that check your T4 and T3 levels (total T4 and T3 and free T4 and T3 can be checked separately). Free T4 or free T3 refers to the level of hormone that is actually servicing your body, rather than the amount of hormone that exists in your body. For more about thyroid testing, see *The Thyroid Sourcebook* and Table 1.1.

Table 1.1 Hypothyroidism at-a-Glance

What You May Notice (listed alphabetically)

- changes in skin pigmentation
- chest pain after physical activity
- constipation
- depression
- difficult-to-manage hair; brittle nails
- difficulty concentrating
- extreme tiredness and slowness
- eyelids that feel "sticky"
- feeling cold
- headaches, problems focusing
- irregular periods or infertility
- loss of interest in sex
- muscle spasms
- shortness of breath
- slow healing, frequent infections
- tingling in hands and feet
- weakness and muscular aches and pains
- weight gain

What Others May Say

- You look pale.
- Your face is puffy.
- Your eyes are swollen.
- Your hair looks/feels coarse or "Are you losing hair?"
- Your voice is husky.
- You snore!
- You used to *love* doing X or Y—why aren't you interested anymore?
- Did you *hear* what I said? (meaning, you can't hear well)

What Your Doctor Should Watch For (listed alphabetically)

- delayed reflexes
- goiter (enlarged thyroid)
- milk leaking from breasts (when you're not breast-feeding)
- muscle weakness
- slowed pulse
- soft abdomen
- tingling or numbness in the hands (sign of carpal tunnel syndrome)

Source: Adapted from Patsy Westcott, *Thyroid Problems: A Practical Guide to Symptoms and Treatment* (London: Thorsons/HarperCollins, 1995), p. 35.

Songs About Hypo Symptoms

Megan Stendebach, a thyroid cancer survivor (diagnosed in 1997), is the "Weird Al" of the thyroid world. Using humor to educate people about hypothyroid symptoms, she has created a funny and warm Web site (www.thyroidcancersongs.com). Reproduced with permission, here are three of her tunes.

My God, I'm a Hypo Boy!

Remember how John Denver made the world seem so simple? Join me now in singing this perky song, *"My God, I'm a Hypo Boy!"*

Well life on the couch is kinda laid back
Ain't much an old hypo boy like me can't hack
It's late to rise and early in the sack
My God, I'm a hypo boy!

Well, a sluggish kinda life never did me no harm
Dozin' on my family and missin' the alarm
My days are all filled with a lazy hypo charm
My God, I'm a hypo boy!

When my nap's all done and sun's settin' low
I pull out my bathrobe and I tie it kinda low
Can't see my feet but they're somewhere down below
My God, I'm a hypo boy!

I'd rather be snorin' all day if I could
But the boss and my wife wouldn't take it very good
So I sleep when I can, work when I should
My God, I'm a hypo boy!

(Chorus)
Well, I got me some Synthroid, maybe too little
When the sun's comin' up I got flab on my middle

Life ain't nothin' but a pesky hypo riddle
My God, I'm a hypo boy!

Well, I would trade my life for diamonds or jewels
I've always been one of those hyper-hungry fools
I'd rather have a middle so my wife kinda drools
My God, I'm a hypo boy!

Hyper folks have energy and stay pretty lean
A lotta hypo people think that's mighty keen
Well, folks, let me tell ya now exactly what I mean
My God! I'm a hypo boy!

(Chorus)
Well I got me some Synthroid, maybe too little
When the sun's comin' up I got flab on my middle
Life ain't nothin' but a pesky hypo riddle
My God, I'm a hypo boy!

Well, they'll fiddle with my dosage till the day I die
Doin' what they can to get my TSH right
Sometimes it's low, sometimes it's high
My God, I'm a hypo boy!

My endo told me, "Son, your dosage is a riddle
Ya oughta feel fine, just as fit as a fiddle.
But you feel like a slug, so we'll raise it just a little."
My God, I'm a hypo boy!

(Chorus)
Well, I got me some Synthroid, maybe too little
When the sun's comin' up I got flab on my middle
Life ain't nothin' but a pesky hypo riddle
My God, I'm a hypo boy!

Oh, My Rear, My Big Fat Rear

Imagine Julie Andrews and the Von Trapp Family Singers going hypothyroid . . .

Oh: my rear, my big fat rear

Hey: this hypo isn't fun

Me: a shame—I'm not myself

Fog: my brain—it cannot run

So: I think I'll go to bed

Blah: to bloat and wallow so

Tea: something to warm my head

That will bring us back to HYpo, HYpo!

(Sing it again!)

The Twelve Weeks of Hypo Hell

OK, kids! It's time for a Sing-Along! This one goes out to all you Hypo-ites out there. Sing it to the tune of "The Twelve Days of Christmas." A-one and a-two . . .

In the first week of hypo hell
my symptoms gave to me
the need for a really great nap.

In the second week of hypo hell
my symptoms gave to me
two migraine headaches,
and the need for a really great nap.

In the third week of hypo hell
my symptoms gave to me
three seafood cravings,
two migraine headaches,
and the need for a really great nap.

In the fourth week of hypo hell
my symptoms gave to me
four bouts of weeping,
three seafood cravings,
two migraine headaches,
and the need for a really great nap.

In the fifth week of hypo hell
my symptoms gave to me
FIVE SLEEPLESS NIGHTS!
Four bouts of weeping,
three seafood cravings,
two migraine headaches,
and the need for a really great nap.

In the sixth week of hypo hell
my symptoms gave to me
six pounds of weight gain,
FIVE SLEEPLESS NIGHTS!
Four bouts of weeping,
three seafood cravings,
two migraine headaches,
and the need for a really great nap.

In the seventh week of hypo hell
my symptoms gave to me
seven days of dry skin,
six pounds of weight gain,
FIVE SLEEPLESS NIGHTS!

Four bouts of weeping,
three seafood cravings,
two migraine headaches,
and the need for a really great nap.

In the eighth week of hypo hell
my symptoms gave to me
eight constipations,
seven days of dry skin,
six pounds of weight gain,
FIVE SLEEPLESS NIGHTS!
Four bouts of weeping,
three seafood cravings,
two migraine headaches,
and the need for a really great nap.

In the ninth week of hypo hell
my symptoms gave to me
nine aching muscles,
eight constipations,
seven days of dry skin,
six pounds of weight gain,
FIVE SLEEPLESS NIGHTS!
Four bouts of weeping,
three seafood cravings,
two migraine headaches,
and the need for a really great nap.

In the tenth week of hypo hell
my symptoms gave to me
ten frozen fingers,
nine aching muscles,
eight constipations,
seven days of dry skin,
six pounds of weight gain,
FIVE SLEEPLESS NIGHTS!

Four bouts of weeping,
three seafood cravings,
two migraine headaches,
and the need for a really great nap.

In the eleventh week of hypo hell
my symptoms gave to me
eleven memory lapses,
and I forget the rest . . .

In the twelfth week of hypo hell
my symptoms gave to me
twelve temper tantrums,
eleven memory lapses,
ten frozen fingers,
nine aching muscles,
eight constipations,
seven days of dry skin,
six pounds of weight gain,
FIVE SLEEPLESS NIGHTS!
Four bouts of weeping,
three seafood cravings,
two migraine headaches,
and THE NEED FOR A REALLY GREAT NAP!!!

2

Are You Sure? Ruling Out Other Health Problems

IF YOU LOOK at the list of symptoms that comprise hypothyroidism in Chapter 1, many are identical to other primary conditions (which may predate, or coincide with, your hypothyroidism). It's always a good idea to rule out other causes for hypo symptoms, such as depression, chronic fatigue syndrome, allergies and environmental sensitivities, or just plain old exhaustion from overwork and stress. Remember: Just because you *have* thyroid disease, it doesn't mean you can't also be suffering from another organic illness or even a situational depression, the symptoms of which are covered below.

Other Causes for Fatigue

Before you immediately blame your thyroid gland for your fatigue, it's important to understand how sick you can feel when you're suffering from just plain old fatigue and stress, due to lack of sleep, overwork, or "garden variety" annoyances. The cure is obvious: Get more sleep and don't work so hard! Trite advice for such trying times! In other words, most of us can't afford the cure if we want to keep paying the mortgage or rent.

Fatigue is one of the most common complaints doctors hear from their patients. It's no big secret that women these days are tired and stressed. Most people have multiple roles, juggling career and family pressures. If you're over forty, chances are you have an ailing parent whom you have to care for on top of your own family.

There is a difference between feeling normal fatigue and chronic fatigue, which is characterized by low energy, lethargy, and flulike symptoms, also signs of hypothyroidism. This section outlines some of the factors responsible for normal fatigue, which can be remedied by making some of the lifestyle changes discussed in Chapter 5.

Sleep Deprivation

People who have demanding jobs that require long hours are often sleep deprived, which can have serious health repercussions. Recent research into sleep deprivation has found not only that it depletes the immune system (depletes you of certain cells needed to destroy viruses and cancerous cells), but it can promote the growth of fat instead of muscle, and may speed up the aging process.

Research also shows that lack of sleep increases levels of the hormone *cortisol*, the "stress hormone." As cortisol rises, muscle-building human-growth hormone and prolactin, a breast-feeding hormone that also helps to protect the immune system, decrease. Normally, cortisol levels should decline while human growth hormone and prolactin should increase during sleep. Cortisol declines prior to sleep because it is the body's way of preparing for sleep. Cortisol normally increases in the morning to make you more alert. Cortisol is released by the adrenal gland in response to stress, and essentially is an "alert" hormone that makes you take action. This is what causes you to be alert in important meetings, "close the sale or deal," or suddenly become incredibly articulate with someone on the phone, after spending five days with two toddlers without any relief. The hormone will subside in the body as the stressful event passes.

A common reason people cut down on their sleep is to get in their "workout time" before their days begin. It's not unusual for many to rise at 5:00 A.M., for example, in order to get their exercise. This, according to sleep experts, only *compromises* health and increases stress. The benefits of the exercise may be canceled out by the detriments of lack of sleep. In the United States, a National Sleep Foundation survey revealed that two out of three people get less than the recommended eight hours of sleep per night, while a third get less than six hours of sleep.

There are two phases of sleep that include rapid eye movement (REM) and non–rapid eye movement. Researchers believe REM sleep is when we dream, an important component in mental health. Non–REM sleep is our deepest sleep when, researchers believe, various hormones are reset and energy stores are replenished.

Right now, roughly 50 percent of people diagnosed with depression get too much REM sleep and not enough deep sleep, which is the "replenishing" sleep.

Aggravating Factors

Caffeine

I'll make this short and sweet: Lots of studies show that caffeine causes anxiety, sleeplessness, and is mildly addictive. It also worsens premenstrual symptoms. Experts now recommend that you consume no more than 400 to 450 mg of caffeine per day, which is equal to two 8-ounce mugs of gourmet coffee or four cups of instant coffee.

Smoking

Many turn to cigarettes to deal with the demands of stress, but people who smoke every day are twice as likely to suffer from depression as people who don't smoke. Smoking will greatly aggravate thyroid problems as well. Nicotine may also be a drug we crave to medicate our depressed moods.

Alcohol

If you tend to have wine or other alcoholic beverages to unwind after a stressful day, be aware that alcohol can interfere with sleep patterns, and is also a depressant. Initially, alcohol may make you tired, and you may think it's a sleeping aid, but it can wake you up later on, making you wide awake at 2:00 A.M., and preventing you from falling back asleep. Naturally, all of this can aggravate stress and fatigue.

Diet

When you're stressed and fatigued, you often don't eat well. By eating properly, and eating a variety of foods—particularly all colors of vegetables—you'll be in better shape to cope. See Chapter 4 for more details.

Chemical Reactions

It's not your imagination that more people are suffering from a range of nondescript aches, pains, and allergies. Exposure to workplace chemicals and toxins are putting many at risk for occupational asthma and allergies, which can lead to chronic fatigue (discussed further on). According to the *Journal of the American Medical Association* (JAMA), at least ten million North Americans suffer from chronic asthma; as much as 15 percent of asthma is directly caused by occupational exposure. One of the most notorious chemicals is toluene diisocyanate (TDI), a chemical used in the plastics and oil industries. It is also found in plants that manufacture boats, recreational vehicles, and electronics.

High-rise office buildings are another source of asthma and allergies due to poor air circulation, causing what is known as "sick building syndrome." Also at risk for asthma and allergies are people who work with animals (the proteins in animal skin and urine can trigger asthma); health care workers who have reactions to natural proteins in rubber latex gloves; and people who work in food plants who inhale dust from cereal protein and flour.

Many notice a significant change in their energy levels and endurance as a result of chronic asthma and allergies from occupational exposure. A ten-year study by the National Institute for Occupational Safety and Health in the United States reveals that asthma is among the leading job-related diseases in the United States and Canada.

Building Supplies

The following materials, common in workplaces, have been cited as hazardous to your health and/or well-being. This doesn't necessarily mean that all are carcinogenic, but many items on this list cause headaches, rashes, and asthmatic symptoms.

- asbestos building materials
- cleaning products and disinfectants
- urea-formaldehyde foam insulation
- adhesives (may contain naphthalene, phenol, ethanol, vinyl chloride, formaldehyde, acrylonitrile, and epoxy, which are toxic substances that release vapors)
- artificial lighting (can cause headaches)
- toners used in copy machines and printers
- particleboard furniture and space dividers
- permanent ink pens and markers (contain acetone, cresol, ethnol, phenol, toluene, and xylene, which are toxic)
- polystyrene cups
- secondhand smoke
- synthetic office carpet (may contain acrylic, polyester, and nylon plastic fibers, and formaldehyde-based finishes, pesticides due to mothproofing for wool only)
- white-out correction fluid (may contain cresol, ethanol, trichloroethlyene, and naphthalene, all toxic chemicals)
- ventilation systems (these can be fodder for mold growth inside ducts; car exhaust when air intakes are placed in parking garages; bacteria from bird feces if birds nest in or around the vents; asbestos fibers and fiberglass)

Multiple Chemical Sensitivity (MCS)

This term was introduced in the early 1990s to explain a wide array of health problems and symptoms that appear to be reactions to chemicals. Among the many different symptoms associated with MCS are depression and chronic fatigue, sleep disturbances, mood swings, and poor concentration. People considered at risk for MCS include those who:

- work or live in energy-sealed buildings
- are exposed to fumes from carpets, pesticides, cleaners, and airborne allergens
- are exposed to industrial chemicals, such as those found in plants that process wood, metal, plastics, paints, and textiles
- are in constant contact with pesticides, fungicides, and fertilizers
- live in high-pollution areas
- work in dry cleaning, hair salons, pest control, printing, or photocopying

Chronic Fatigue Syndrome

Seventy percent of all people who suffer from chronic fatigue are women under the age of forty-five. Many may be misdiagnosed with a thyroid condition or depression. Chronic fatigue syndrome (CFS) has been around longer than you might think. In 1843, for example, a curious condition called "fibrositis" was described by doctors, characterized by similar symptoms now seen in *fibromyalgia* (chronic muscle and joint aches and pains) and *chronic fatigue syndrome* (symptoms of fibromyalgia, accompanied by flulike symptoms and extreme fatigue—see further on). The term *rheumatism*, an outdated label, was frequently used as well to describe various aches and pains with no specific or identifiable origin.

In the late 1970s and early 1980s, a mysterious virus known as Epstein-Barr was being diagnosed in thousands of young, upwardly mobile professionals—at the time known as "Yuppies"—from the baby boom generation. People were calling this condition the "Yuppie flu," the "Yuppie virus," "Yuppie syndrome," and "burnout" syndrome.

Many medical professionals were stumped by it, and many disregarded it as a phantom illness or a psychosomatic illness. Because so many women were dismissed by their doctors as hypochondriacs, or not believed to be ill or fatigued, the physical symptoms triggered self-doubts, feelings of low self-esteem, self-loathing, and so on, which often triggered depression. But even with the most sensitive medical attention, depression seems to go hand in hand with CFS simply because the disorder leaves so many sufferers at home in bed, isolated from the active lifestyle so many CFS sufferers once had. In other words, some believe that in the case of CFS, depression is a normal response to "feeling lousy" every day of your life! It's another example of the "if you weren't depressed, you'd be crazy" adage I use in this book.

A lot of people with CFS were also misdiagnosed with various other diseases that shared some of the symptoms we now define as CFS. These diseases included mononucleosis, multiple sclerosis, and HIV-related illnesses (once called AIDS-related complex, or ARC), Lyme disease, post-polio syndrome, and lupus. If you were diagnosed with *any* of the above diseases, please take a look at the established symptom criteria for CFS that follow. You may have been misdiagnosed, which is an extremely common scenario.

In the early 1980s, two physicians in Nevada who treated a number of patients who shared this curious condition (after a nasty winter flu had hit the region) identified it as "chronic fatigue syndrome." This label is perhaps most accurate, and the one that has stuck.

There are other names for CFS, such as the U.K. label ME, which stands for myalgic encephalomyelitis, as well as post viral fatigue syndrome. CFS is also known as chronic fatigue immune deficiency syndrome (CFIDS), because it's now believed that CFS sufferers are immune suppressed, although this is still in debate. But for the purposes of this chapter, I'll refer to the simpler label that seems to tell it like it is: chronic fatigue syndrome.

The Symptoms of CFS

The term *chronic fatigue syndrome* refers to a *collection* of ill-health symptoms (not just one or two), the most identifiable of which are fatigue and flulike aches and pains.

It wasn't until 1994 that an official definition of chronic fatigue syndrome (CFS) was published in the *Annals of Internal Medicine*. The Centers for Disease Control (CDC) have since published official symptoms of CFS, too. Although many physicians feel the following list of symptoms is limiting and requires some expansion for accuracy, as of this writing the official defining symptoms of CFS include:

1. *An unexplained fatigue that is "new."* In other words, you've previously felt fine and have only noticed in the past six months or so that you're always fatigued, no matter *how* much rest you get. The fatigue is also debilitating for you; you're not as productive at work, and it interferes with normal activities that may be social, personal, or academic. You've also noticed poor memory or concentration, which affects your activities and performance.

2. In addition to this fatigue, you have four or more of the following, which have persisted for at least six months:

- sore throat
- mild or low-grade fever
- tenderness in the neck and underarm area (where you have lymph nodes that may be swollen, causing tenderness)
- muscle pain (called myalgia)
- pain along the nerve of a joint, without redness or swelling
- a strange and new kind of headache you've never suffered from before
- you sleep but wake up unrefreshed (a sign of insufficient amounts of non-REM sleep, as discussed earlier)
- you feel tired, weak, and generally unwell for a good twenty-four hours after you've had even moderate exercise (see below)

3. *Poor exercise tolerance.* Some CFS experts feel that "poor exercise tolerance" (even modest exercise is followed by such exhaustion and malaise, you can't tolerate it) is perhaps the hallmark symptom of

CFS. Research into CFS has uncovered that there is indeed a biological reason for this that has to do with a deficient flow of oxygen and energy to your cells during exercise. Normally, oxygen increases in our bodies with exercise. In CFS sufferers, the opposite has been found: Oxygen seems to decrease with exercise, which may explain a lot! Without oxygen during exercise, various "poisons" (accumulated substances we produce naturally, such as lactic acid, magnesium, and others) can build up and reduce the efficiency of our tissues and organs. Why this is happening remains to be discovered, while the issue of whether this is happening at all still needs to be confirmed and further documented, according to many other scientists.

Fibromyalgia Versus CFS

Fibromyalgia is a soft-tissue disorder that causes you to hurt all over— all the time. It appears to be a condition that is triggered and/or aggravated by stress. If you notice fatigue and more general aches and pains, this suggests CFS. If you notice *primarily* joint and muscle pains, *accompanied* by fatigue, this suggests fibromyalgia. It is sometimes considered to be an offshoot of arthritis, and it's not unusual to be misdiagnosed with rheumatoid arthritis. Headaches, morning stiffness, and intolerance to cold, damp weather are common complaints with fibromyalgia. It's also common to suffer from irritable bowel syndrome or bladder problems with this disorder.

Causes of CFS

There is no official, known cause of CFS. But several theories suggest viral agents infecting the population (the book *Osler's Web* implies this, and further speculates that there is an active government cover-up of such viruses). Others believe the cause to be airborne environmental toxins and poisons, which can impact the immune system.

Some CFS sufferers have an impaired immune system, similar to what happens with HIV infection. This suggests there *may* be some viral agent(s) at work. But other CFS sufferers have an overactive immune system, suggesting that CFS may be an autoimmune condition, meaning that your immune system manufactures antibodies that attack your body's own tissues. Autoimmune diseases are triggered by stress. The pain and inflammation many CFS sufferers report is more likely due to the overactive immune system; the flulike malaise and fatigue is more likely due to an underactive immune system. This is why CFS continues to remain a mystery to researchers. When a body is poisoned by environmental toxins, however, it's possible that different toxins can trigger different reactions by the immune system, which may explain the paradox. Gulf War syndrome, for example, is characterized by a wide array of symptoms. Different bodies may react differently to the same toxin, too.

Stress appears to be a major trigger of CFS. When we are under stress, our bodies produce the hormone *adrenaline*, which increases our heart rate, blood flow, blood pressure, and so on. Adrenaline may aggravate the inflammation and pain many CFS and fibromyalgia sufferers experience.

Some experts who treat CFS and fibromyalgia believe that a lack of non-REM sleep may be a factor in this disorder. Some have gone on record to say that chronic fatigue syndrome is really a sleep-related disorder. One Canadian study deliberately deprived a group of medical students of non-REM sleep over a period of several nights. Within the next few days, each of the study participants developed symptoms of CFS and/or fibromyalgia.

Treatments

Most experts agree that CFS is an environmental illness, triggered by stress. Diet and lifestyle modification appears to be an effective way to treat CFS, as certain "trigger foods"—foods that typically trigger allergies or fungal infections with the fungus *Candida albicans* (processed foods, foods high in sugar or yeast, and so on)—are eliminated and replaced with more nutritious, vitamin-packed, organic foods. Since so many CFS sufferers have *Candida*, adjusting the diet is a logical first step. *Candida* is a parasite that normally inhabits our digestive tract. This parasite can overgrow and spread to other places in the body, damaging the immune system.

Often a move to a cleaner environment is useful (changing jobs or telecommuting if you believe you're being exposed to workplace toxins; moving from an urban center to a suburb or rural area).

"Downshifting," a term coined to describe people who simplify their lifestyles, shedding the urban "noise and toys," often works wonders to shed some stress, which can often improve CFS. This may involve moving to a smaller home with a lower monthly payment, leaving a job, buying that farm you've always wanted, or blowing your "retirement money" and taking a long trip.

CFS experts and fellow sufferers caution you about taking antidepressants—often the first thing a medical doctor will prescribe. Since antidepressants have many side effects that can aggravate CFS symptoms, they are reportedly not the best solution as a "first-line" treatment for CFS. The general advice is to try cleaning up the diet and lifestyle first and see if your symptoms improve. Symptoms of depression in CFS often resolve when you start to feel a little better physically, and get out of the house!

Numerous alternative therapies are reported to work with CFS. Many of these organizations have Web sites, monthly newsletters with the "latest" treatment trends, and so on. I hesitate, as of this writing, to recommend much of what I came across in my research because it is simply not yet substantiated. But like so many herbs and alternative therapies, ranging from glucosamine sulphate (for arthritis) to St. John's wort, just because they're not proven in traditional scientific studies doesn't mean they don't work. Time will tell, as well as word of mouth. To date, however, diet modification is the most effective treatment CFS experts recommend, along with cognitive therapy, a type of counseling that helps you to "shift" your thinking or focus.

Ruling Out Depression

Depression and hypothyroidism crash into each other all the time. For example, roughly 15 percent of those diagnosed with depression (which now affects about 20 percent of the general population) suffer from hypothyroidism. But again, just because you have a thyroid problem does not mean it is the sole cause for depression symptoms. You should rule out other causes for depression if you can, which will make managing hypothyroidism a little easier, too. Table 2.1 will help you cross-check depression symptoms against symptoms of hypothyroidism. Many of you may benefit from my book *50 Ways to Prevent Depression.* Women may also benefit from reading my books *Women and Depression* and *Women and Passion.* To rule out other causes for depression, let's review the symptoms of depression.

Signs of Depression

Depression is clinically known as a "mood disorder." It's impossible to define what a "normal mood" is since we all have such complex personalities, and we each exhibit different moods throughout a given week, or even a given day. But it's not impossible for *you* to define what a "normal" mood is for *you. You* know how you feel when you're functional: you're eating, sleeping, interacting with friends and family, being productive, active, and generally interested in the daily goings-on in life. Well, depression is when you feel you've *lost* the ability to function for a prolonged period of time, or you may be functioning at a reasonable level to the outside world but you've lost *interest* in participating in life.

One bad day, or even a bad week (which will usually be made up of some "relief time" where you can laugh at something or take pleasure in something), from time to time is not a sign that you're depressed. Feeling you've lost the ability to function as you *normally* do, all day, every day, for a period of at least two weeks, may be a sign that you're depressed. The symptoms of depression can vary from person to person, but can include some or all of the symptoms listed in Table 2.1.

Anhedonia: When Nothing Gives You Pleasure

One of the most telling signs of depression is a loss of interest in activities that used to excite you, enthuse you, or give you pleasure. This is known as anhedonia, derived from the word *hedonism* (meaning "phi-

Table 2.1 Symptoms of Major Depression, Hypothyroidism, and Hyperthyroidism

The following symptoms can indicate major depression as well as hypo- or hyperthyroidism. Symptoms in **bold** represent signs of hypothyroidism; symptoms in *italics* represent signs of hyperthyroidism:

- **feelings of sadness and/or "empty mood"**
- *difficulty sleeping (usually waking up frequently in the middle of the night)*
- **loss of energy and feelings of fatigue and lethargy**
- **change in appetite (usually a loss of appetite)**
- **difficulty thinking, concentrating, or making decisions (see section further on)**
- **loss of interest in formerly pleasurable activities, including sex**
- *anxiety or panic attacks (characterized by racing heart)*
- obsessing over negative experiences or thoughts
- feeling guilty, worthless, hopeless, or helpless
- *feeling restless and irritable*
- thinking about death or suicide

losophy of pleasure"); a "hedonist" is a person who indulges her every pleasure without considering (or caring about) the consequences. Anhedonia simply means "no pleasure."

Different people have different ways of expressing anhedonia. You might tell your friends, for example, that you don't "have any desire" to do X or Y; you can't "get motivated"; or X or Y just doesn't "hold your interest or attention." You may also notice that the sense of satisfaction from a job well done is simply gone, which is particularly debilitating in the workplace or in a place of learning. For example, artists (photographers, painters, writers, and others) may find the passion has gone out of their work.

Many of the symptoms of depression hinge on this "loss of pleasure" symptom. One of the reasons weight loss is so common in depression (typically, people may notice as much as a 10-pound drop in weight) is because food no longer gives them pleasure, or cooking no longer gives them pleasure. The sense of satisfaction we get from having a clean home or clean kitchen may also disappear. Tackling cleaning up our kitchens in order to prepare food may be too taxing, contributing to a lack of interest in food.

Of course, gaining weight is not unusual either: 10 pounds in the opposite direction can occur, too. This is often due to poor nutrition: Because we're not eating properly, we fill up on snack foods, or high-calorie, low-nutrient foods because we're not motivated to eat or prepare well-balanced meals. Weight gain may also come from a loss of interest in physical activities such as exercising, sports, or a dozen other things that keep us active when we're feeling "ourselves."

A loss of interest in sex aggravates matters if we are in a sexual relationship with someone. Again, the decreased desire for sex stems from general anhedonia.

When You Can't Think Clearly

Another debilitating feature of depression is finding that you simply can't concentrate or think clearly. You feel scattered, disorganized, and unable to prioritize. This usually hits hardest in the workplace or a center of learning, and can severely impair your performance on the job. You may miss important deadlines, important meetings, or find you can't focus when you *do* go to meetings. When you can't think clearly, you can be overwhelmed with feelings of helplessness or hopelessness. "I can't even perform a simple task such as X anymore" may dominate your thoughts, while you become more disillusioned with your dwindling productivity.

When You Can't Sleep

The typical sleep pattern of a depressed person is to go to bed at the normal time, only to wake up around two in the morning and find that she can't get back to sleep. Endless hours are spent watching infomercials to pass the time, or simply tossing and turning, usually obsessing over negative experiences or thoughts. Lack of sleep affects our ability to function, and leads to increased irritability, lack of energy, and fatigue. Insomnia, by itself, is not a sign of depression, but when you look at depression as a package of symptoms, the inability to fall or stay asleep can aggravate all your other symptoms. In some cases, people who are depressed will oversleep, requiring ten to twelve hours of sleep every night.

These symptoms refer to major depression, the "cold and flu" of mood disorders for psychiatrists.

Managing Depression

When you're suffering from the symptoms of depression, the first order of business is to get you back to your functioning self again. Long-term strategies to prevent a recurrence will vary, depending on the circumstances of your depression, and the type of depression you're suffering from. There is no one way to manage depression since different things work for different people. Less invasive solutions involve finding someone to talk to, in counseling or psychotherapy. Talk therapy may work best in combination with antidepressants or herbal remedies such as St. John's wort.

Herbal Remedies

In 1997, the American Psychiatric Association stated that the herb St. John's wort can be started as a "first-line" treatment for mild to moderate depression. The herb is named after St. John, the patron saint of nurses, while "wort" is simply Old English for "plant." It is essentially the "nurses' plant." St. John's wort can apparently work as well in many people as a prescription antidepressant because it relieves stress. It is also known to relieve other stress-related problems, including gastrointestinal ailments.

St. John's wort has been used successfully for years throughout Europe, while studies show that it can do the same job as antidepressants without as many side effects.

Antidepressants

Antidepressants work on your brain chemistry. There are several types of prescription antidepressants, known as heterocyclics, monamine oxidase inhibitors (MAOIs), and selective serotonin reuptake inhibitors

(SSRIs). A subtype of SSRIs, called MSRIs, which stands for mixed serotonin reuptake inhibitors, is also popular, and includes serotonin-norepinephrine reuptake inhibitors (SNRIs). There are other kinds of antidepressants as well.

Long-Term Solutions

Preventing a recurrence of a depressive episode involves prolonged therapy: long-term counseling and/or psychotherapy instead of short-term; long-term talk therapy in combination with medications or herbs; and lifestyle changes (ranging from stress reduction techniques to dramatic changes involving residence, jobs, and interpersonal relationships). Since long-term solutions often involve making dramatic changes in your lifestyle, which can take a *long time* to come to terms with, or to implement, counseling is often a key component in managing depression.

Seasonal Affective Disorder (SAD)

Symptoms of hypothyroidism have a lot in common with symptoms of seasonal affective disorder (SAD), a "blue mood" triggered by changes in seasons. The typical person with SAD will notice that she sleeps too much and eats too much (thereby gaining weight). Then she begins to "wake up" in the spring, and can even be slightly manic (known as hypomanic). Occasionally, the reverse occurs, and the depression comes on during the summer months instead, when the symptoms of major depression present themselves. Some of this may be related to extreme discomfort in humid, hot weather, inability to sleep as a result, increased pollutants in the air, and all the other miseries of humid, hot, urban summers.

SAD strikes many people in their twenties and thirties, and is seen more in regions at higher latitudes. Light at the end of the tunnel is in sight for women with SAD—literally. Bright light is the treatment, which you should discuss with your doctor.

Other Causes for Weight Gain

Hypothyroidism can aggravate a *preexisting* weight problem, which is usually the more serious consequence of a thyroid condition for most people. If you weigh 20 percent more than your ideal weight for your height and age, you are technically considered obese. When obesity is due to hypothyroidism, most people will find that they return to their normal weight when their hypothyroidism is treated. Feeling tired and low in energy, a symptom of hypothyroidism, can cause you to crave carbohydrates and quick-energy foods, which are higher in fat and calories. When you're hypothyroid, your activity levels will decrease as a result of your fatigue, which can also lead to weight gain. The craving for carbohydrates is caused by a desire for energy. Consuming carbohydrates produces an initial "rush" of energy, but then it is followed by a tremendous "crash," sometimes known as postprandial depression (or postmeal depression), exacerbating or contributing to hypothyroid-induced depression. Even in people with normal thyroid function, depression can cause cravings for simple carbohydrates, such as sugars and sweets. Many women will notice that they are not craving food at all, but are still gaining weight. Some of the weight gain is bloating from constipation. Increasing fluid intake and fiber will help the problem.

Obviously cutting down on fat (see Chapter 4) will also help. But the problem for most who are battling both obesity and hypothyroidism is that the weight problem often predates the thyroid problem, indicating that there are other factors involved in their weight gain. Stack a thyroid problem on top of that, and it may exacerbate all kinds of other behaviors that led to the initial weight gain, as well as aggravate risks associated with obesity in general, such as Type 2 diabetes, heart disease, or stroke. This section therefore examines other factors that lead to obesity so you can help to "weed out" nonthyroid and thyroid-related reasons for your weight gain.

Chronic Dieting

Many obese people say that they've "dieted themselves up" to their present weight. Indeed, the road to obesity is paved with chronic dieting. It is estimated that at least 50 percent of all North American women are dieting at any given time, while one-third of North American dieters initiate a diet at least once a month. The very act of dieting in your teens and twenties can predispose you to obesity in your thirties, forties, and beyond. This occurs because most people "crash and burn" instead of eating sensibly. In other words, they're chronic dieters.

The crash-and-burn approach to diet is what we do when we want to lose a specific number of pounds for a particular occasion or outfit. The pattern is to starve for a few days and then eat what we normally do. Or, we eat only certain foods (such as celery and grapefruit) for a number of days and then eat normally after we've lost the weight. Most of these diets do not incorporate exercise, which means that we burn up some of our muscle as well as fat. Then, when we eat normally, we gain only fat. And over the years that fat simply grows fatter. The bottom line is that when there is more fat on your body than muscle, you cannot burn calories as efficiently. It is the muscle that makes it possible to burn calories. Diet it away, and you diet away your ability to burn fat.

If starvation is involved in our trying to lose weight, our bodies become more efficient at getting fat. Starvation triggers an intelligence in the metabolism; our body suddenly thinks we're living in a war zone and goes into "superefficient nomadic mode," not realizing that we're living in North America. So, when we return to our normal caloric intake, or even a *lower*-than-normal caloric intake after we've starved ourselves, *we gain more weight*. Our bodies say: "Oh look—food! Better store that as fat for the next famine." Some researchers believe that starvation diets slow down our metabolic rates far below normal so that weight gain becomes more rapid after each starvation episode.

This cycle of crash or starvation dieting is known as the yo-yo diet syndrome, the subject of thousands of articles in magazines throughout the past twenty years. Breaking the pattern sounds easy: Combine exercise with a sensible diet. But it's not that easy if you've led a sedentary life most of your adult years. Ninety-five percent of the people who go on a diet gain back the weight they lost, as well as extra weight, within two years. As discussed further on, the failure often lies in psychological and behavioral factors. We have to understand why we need to eat before we can eat less. The best way to break the yo-yo diet pattern is to educate our children early about food habits and appropriate body weight. Experts say that unless you are significantly overweight to begin with or have a medical condition, *don't diet.* Just eat well.

But If You're Gonna Diet . . .

A recent study suggests that prepackaged balanced meals can help you stick to a meal plan more easily if you do indeed need to lose weight. Therefore, plan your meals in advance with a nutritionist and try to prefreeze or refrigerate them. This will help curb impulse eating. If you're contemplating a diet, you should also consider the following:

- What is a reasonable weight for you, given your genetic makeup, family history, age, and culture? A smaller weight loss in some people can produce dramatic effects.
- Aim to lose weight at a slower rate. Too much too fast will probably lead to gaining it all back.
- Incorporate exercise into your routine, particularly activities that build muscle mass.
- Eat your vitamins. Many of the popular North American diets of the 1980s, for example, were nutritionally inadequate (the Beverly Hills Diet contained 0 percent of the U.S. recommendation for vitamin B_{12}).

Compulsive Eating

The physical symptoms associated with hypothyroidism can exacerbate compulsive eating behavior that predates the hypothyroidism. The craving for carbohydrates (see above) can also wreak havoc on preexisting eating behaviors. When we hear "eating disorder," we usually think about anorexia or bulimia. There are many people, however, who binge without purging. This is also known as binge eating disorder (aka compulsive overeating). In this case, the bingeing is still an announcement to the world that "I'm out of control." Someone who purges is hiding his/her lack of control. Someone who binges and never purges is *advertising* his/her lack of control. The purger is passively asking for help; the binger who doesn't purge is aggressively asking for help. It's the same disease with a different result.

But there is one more layer when it comes to compulsive overeating, which is considered to be controversial, and often rejected by the overeater: the desire to get fat is often behind the compulsion. Many people who overeat insist that fat is a consequence of eating food, not a *goal*. Many therapists who deal with overeating disagree, and believe that if people admit that they have an emotional interest in actually being large, they may be much closer to stopping their compulsion to eat.

Furthermore, many who eat compulsively do not recognize that they are doing so. The following is a typical profile of a compulsive eater:

- eating when you're not hungry
- feeling out of control when you're around food, either trying to resist it or gorging on it
- spending a lot of time thinking/worrying about food and your weight
- always desperate to try another diet that promises results
- obsessed with what you can or will eat, or *have* eaten
- eating in secret or with "eating friends"
- appearing in public to be a professional dieter who's in control
- buying cakes or pies as "gifts" and having them wrapped to hide the fact that they're for you
- having a "pristine" kitchen with only the "right" foods
- feeling either out-of-control with food (compulsive eating) or imprisoned by it (dieting)
- feeling temporary relief by "not eating"
- feelings of self-loathing and shame
- hating your own body
- looking forward with pleasure and anticipation to the time when you can eat alone
- feeling unhappy because of your eating behavior

Biological Causes of Obesity

Since diet and lifestyle changes are so difficult, there is an interest in finding genetic causes for obesity. That would mean that obesity is *beyond our control*—and something we've inherited, which would probably be comforting for many people. Now that we have completed the Human Genome Project, a project that maps every gene in the human body, research into the "obesity gene" or "fat gene" is under way. But few scientists believe that obesity is *simply* genetic. In other words, there are so many environmental and social factors that can "trip" the obesity "switch" that finding a specific gene for obesity is about as worthwhile as finding the "anger gene" or "crime gene."

There are also many theories surrounding the function of fat cells. Are some people genetically programmed to have more, or "fatter," fat cells than others? No answers here, yet.

What about the brain and obesity? Some propose that obesity is "all in the head" and has something to do with the hypothalamus (a part of the brain that controls messages to other parts of the body) somehow malfunctioning when it comes to sending the body the message "I'm full." It's believed that the hypothalamus may control "satiation messages."

To other researchers, the problem has to do with some sort of defect in the body that doesn't recognize hunger cues or satiation cues, but the studies in this area are not conclusive.

What About the Fat Hormone?

A study reported in a 1997 issue of *Nature Medicine* showed that people with low levels of the hormone leptin may be prone to weight gain. In this study, people who gained an average of 50 pounds over three years started out with lower leptin levels than people who maintained their weight over the same period. Therefore, this study may form the basis for treating obesity with leptin. Experts speculate that 10 percent of all obesity may be due to a leptin resistance. Leptin is made by fat cells and apparently sends messages to the brain about how much fat our bodies are carrying. Like other hormones, it's thought that leptin has a stimulating action that acts as a thermostat of sorts. In mice, adequate amounts of leptin somehow signaled the mouse to become more active and eat less, while too little leptin signaled the mouse to eat more while becoming less active.

Interestingly, Pima Indians, who are prone to obesity, were shown to have roughly one-third less leptin in blood analyses. Human studies of injecting leptin to treat obesity are in the works right now, but to date have not been shown to be effective.

Obesity Drugs

One of the oldest and most misused weight loss drugs around is, in fact, thyroid hormone. Until at least 1980, many women battling a weight problem were prescribed thyroid hormone by some doctors. When this practice was banned, anecdotal evidence shows that women with legitimate thyroid disorders were giving their pills out to friends or family members who wanted them for weight control. Taking thyroid hormone when you have a normal, functioning thyroid will cause you to become hyperthyroid, which can have serious consequences for your heart (see Chapter 1) if hyperthyroidism is prolonged.

In the not-too-distant past, amphetamines, or "speed," were often widely peddled to people battling weight problems, but they are dangerous too, and can put your health at risk.

Antiobesity Pills

The U.S. government recently approved an antiobesity pill that blocks the absorption of almost one-third of the fat people eat. One of the side effects of this new prescription drug, called orlistat (Xenical), is rather embarrassing diarrhea each time you eat fatty foods. To avoid the drug's side effects, simply avoid fat! The pill can also decrease absorption of vitamin D and other important nutrients.

Orlistat is the first drug to fight obesity through the intestine instead of the brain. Taken with each meal, it binds to certain pancreatic enzymes to block the digestion of 30 percent of the fat you ingest. How it affects the pancreas in the long term is not known. Combined with a sensible diet, people on orlistat lost more weight than those not on orlistat. This drug is not intended for people who need to lose a few pounds; it is designed for medically obese people. (Orlistat was also found to lower cholesterol, blood pressure, and blood sugar levels.)

Another obesity drug, sibutramine, was approved for use in 2001. Sibutramine is meant for people whose body mass index (BMI) registers at 27 or higher. This is generally people who weigh more than 20 percent of their ideal weight. To calculate your BMI, you can visit www.4meridia.com.

Anyone with high blood pressure is cautioned against taking sibutramine, because sibutramine can significantly raise your blood pressure. If you're being treated for thyroid disease of any kind, are taking medications for depression, seizures, glaucoma, osteoporosis, gallbladder disease, liver disease, heart disease or stroke prevention, kidney disease, migraines, or Parkinson's disease, you are also cautioned against taking sibutramine, and instructed to discuss with your doctor whether the drug is safe. Also, many nutritional supplements, such as tryptophan, are not recommended with sibutramine, so please disclose to your doctor all nonprescription, over-the-counter medications as well as all herbal and nutritional substances you're taking if you're considering sibutramine. One of the most controversial antiobesity therapies was the use of Fenfluramine and Phentermine (Fen/Phen). Both drugs were approved for use individually more than twenty years ago, but since 1992, doctors tended to prescribe them together for long-term management of obesity. In 1996, U.S. doctors wrote a total of eighteen million monthly prescriptions for Fen/Phen. And many of the prescriptions were issued to people who were not obese. This is known as "off-label" prescribing. In July 1997, the U.S. Food and Drug Administration, along with researchers at the Mayo Clinic and the Mayo Foundation, made a joint announcement warning doctors that Fen/Phen can cause heart disease. On September 15, 1997, "Fen" was taken off the market. The Fen/Phen lesson: Diet and lifestyle modifications are still the best pathway to wellness. (More bad news has surfaced about Fen/Phen wreaking havoc on serotonin levels, which only reinforces the Fen/Phen lesson.)

For more information about overcoming weight gain as a result of hypothyroidism or a preexisting weight problem, see "The Hypothyroid Diet" in Chapter 4.

3

When Your Doctor Says "Take a Pill"

LET'S ASSUME YOU know why you're hypothyroid (see Chapter 1), and you've ruled out other causes for your symptoms, or aggravating conditions. You will be told to "take a pill" unless there's a good reason *not* to treat you immediately for your hypothyroidism (for example, are you receiving radioactive iodine for Graves' disease or thyroid cancer?; see *The Thyroid Sourcebook, 4th edition*). Mary Shomon, author of *Living Well with Hypothyroidism*, makes an important point about thyroid hormone medication: *one pill does not fit all.* Many people like myself have been healthy, balanced, and happy with our thyroid hormone pills (I have been taking a brand-name synthetic thyroid hormone pill faithfully each morning since 1983 after my bout with thyroid cancer at age twenty). But many others like Mary Shomon have *not* been feeling well on their thyroid hormone pill, and have had to investigate alternatives to the "standard issue" synthetically produced thyroxine (aka T4), which goes by the generic drug name of levothyroxine sodium. This chapter looks at all the issues surrounding thyroid hormone medication. If you're reading this chapter and are not feeling well, I urge you to also look at the chapters following this, designed to optimize your health on thyroid hormone medication. "The Hypothyroid Diet" (Chapter 4), "The Hypothyroid Active Living Program" (Chapter 5), and "The Hypothyroid Herbal and Wellness Program"

(Chapter 6) are filled with tools to maximize your health and help you to feel well again.

What Is Thyroid Medication?

When you're taking thyroid medication, you're either on thyroid replacement hormone for life to compensate for a hypothyroid condition (often the result of treatment for hyperthyroidism or thyroid cancer), or you're taking antithyroid medication to control hyperthyroidism (for more information on this, see *The Thyroid Sourcebook, 4th edition*).

Thyroid Hormone Replacement

In the United States, more than fifteen million prescriptions of thyroid hormone are sold annually. Even if only part of your thyroid gland is surgically removed, thyroid hormone replacement may be prescribed.

A prescription for thyroid hormone replacement pills costs anywhere from $15 to $30 for a three-month supply, depending on the brand. The most common replacement hormone is levothyroxine sodium, a synthetically produced version of thyroxine, or T4. This is considered the first-line therapy for thyroid replacement hormone, but that doesn't mean it will be the right fit for you. There are other forms of hormone you can get (see further on).

Levothyroxine sodium comes color-coded. Each color represents a different strength, depending on the brand. Thyroid hormone replacement pills are color-coded to improve what pharmacists refer to as "patient compliance." When each dosage comes in a different color, it's much easier for patients to say "I'm taking the pink pill" instead of "I'm taking 112 micrograms," for example. See Table 3.1 for a complete list of colors, dosage strengths, and suggested guidelines according to weight. If you have a problem with dyes used to color the pills, most brands offer their 50-microgram strength as a plain white pill, without dye. Pharmaceutical manufacturers recommend that you ask your doctor to prescribe your thyroid hormone replacement in increments of the white pill (such as 50 micrograms) if you're expe-

Table 3.1 The United Colors of Thyroid Hormone Replacement Pills

Thyroid hormone replacement is color-coded by dose. Dose is usually determined by weight, unless the goal is TSH suppression, or there are other medical conditions at work. Below is a *general* guideline only, in micrograms, assuming approximately 1.6 micrograms of thyroid hormone replacement daily for every kilogram of adult body weight. After age 65, expect your dosage to decrease by about 10 percent. Eltroxin is available only in Canada. Levoxyl and Levothroid are available only in the United States. Please note that this table does not represent all brands of thyroid hormone sold in North America and is intended as a very general guideline only.

Color	Dosage	Brands	Weight Range
orange	25	Synthroid/Levoxyl/Levothroid	16–23 kg/30–50 lbs
white	50	Synthroid/Levoxyl/Levothroid/Eltroxin	24–39 kg/51–87 lbs
violet	75	Synthroid	40–51 kg/88–112 lbs
purple	75	Levoxyl	Same
gray	75	Levothroid	Same
olive	88	Synthroid/Levoxyl	52–59 kg/113–131 lbs
mint green	88	Levothroid	Same
yellow	100	Synthroid/Levoxyl/Levothroid/Eltroxin	60–66 kg/132–146 lbs
rose	112	Synthroid/Levoxyl/Levothroid	67–74 kg/147–163 lbs
brown	125	Synthroid/Levoxyl	75–86 kg/164–190 lbs
purple	125	Levothroid	Same
dark blue	137	Levoxyl	82–91 kg/180–200 lbs
blue	137	Levothroid	Same
light blue	150	Synthroid/Levoxyl/Levothroid/Eltroxin	87–101 kg/191–225 lbs
lilac	175	Synthroid	Special cases
turquoise	175	Levoxyl/Levothroid	Same
pink	200	Synthroid/Levoxyl/Levothroid/Eltroxin	Same
green	300	Synthroid/Levoxyl/Levothroid/Eltroxin	Same

Sources: 1. "Solving the Puzzle of Hypothyroidism." Physician literature, supplied by Knoll Pharma Inc., 1995. 2. Levoxyl Prescribing Information, Daniels Pharmaceuticals, Inc., 1994. 3. Levothroid Prescribing Information, Forest Pharmaceuticals, Inc., 1995. 4. Eltroxin Prescribing Information, GlaxoWellcome, Inc., 1995.

riencing a reaction. See "What's In This Stuff, Anyway?" (page 59) for more information.

If you're taking multivitamin pills or iron supplements, such as ferrous sulphate, take your thyroid hormone pill at least two hours in advance. Iron appears to bind to thyroid hormone, making less of it available for absorption by your body.

Other Forms of Thyroid Hormone

Thyroid hormone has come a long way. In the 1890s, medical textbooks gave "recipes" for preparing animal thyroid glands as a treatment for thyroid patients. You were likely to have "fried, minced thyroid" served with bread and currant jelly for breakfast. A few decades back, the first form of thyroid replacement hormone used was dessicated thyroid hormone, which was composed of dried animal thyroid hormone. Unlike the synthetic hormone today, dried animal thyroid hormone was a mixture of T4 and T3, and no two mixtures of dessicated thyroid hormone were alike. For example, one pill may have contained three parts T3 and one part T4, while another contained the reverse. As a result, although dessicated thyroid hormone worked, it was jarring to other bodily systems since it was crudely produced. Today, you can get a synthetic combination of T3/T4, which is sold in the United States under the brand name Thyrolar. Natural thyroid hormone, made from pigs' thyroid glands, is still sold under the brand names Armour Thyroid, Naturethroid, and Westhroid.

The Right Dosage

If you're on too high a dosage of thyroid hormone (no matter what brand), you'll develop all the classic symptoms of hyperthyroidism (see Table 3.2). If this happens, notify your doctor; he or she will adjust your dosage accordingly. The correct dosage of thyroid hormone is determined by a normal TSH reading and other blood tests (see Chapter 1).

After treatment for hyperthyroidism, the average dose for levothyroxine sodium is around 112 micrograms. Most people will be able to find the right dose in the seven or eight dosage strengths various brands offer, which range between 50 and 150 micrograms. The average daily dose after thyroid cancer treatment ranges from 100 to 200 micrograms.

If You've Had Thyroid Cancer

The appropriate thyroid hormone replacement dosage is slightly different for thyroid cancer patients. That's because the goals of therapy are a little different. Any microscopic piece of thyroid tissue in your body will

Table 3.2 Hyperthyroidism at-a-Glance

If you're on too high a dosage of thyroid hormone medication, you could become hyperthyroid. Here's a quick checklist of hyperthyroid symptoms to watch for.

What You May Notice
(listed alphabetically)

- anxiety and irritability
- changes in menstrual cycle, such as no periods, longer, or shorter cycle
- dry, thin skin that turns red more easily
- enlarged thyroid
- eye problems or irritations
- feeling hot all the time
- hair loss
- increased appetite
- increased sex drive
- increased sweating
- insomnia
- muscle weakness
- palpitations
- staring eyes
- warm, moist palms
- weight loss

What Others May Say

- You're moody.
- You're so talkative lately!
- You seem agitated.
- Your neck looks swollen .
- Why are you staring like that? (i.e., your eyes have a "staring" look)
- You've lost weight.
- You're shaking.

What Your Doctor Should Look For
(listed alphabetically)

- fast pulse
- irregular heartbeat (atrial fibrilation)
- low blood pressure
- quick reflexes
- tremor

Source: Adapted from Patsy Westcott, *Thyroid Problems: A Practical Guide to Symptoms and Treatment* (London: Thorsons/HarperCollins, 1995), p. 45.

be stimulated by TSH. If that thyroid tissue is cancerous, then TSH may stimulate cancerous tissue to grow. In your case, the trick is to find a high enough dosage to suppress your TSH, which means that your T4 readings will be *higher* than in just "plain 'ol hypothyroid" patients. *But* you need not suffer any hyperthyroid symptoms. TSH suppression can be accomplished with one of the precise doses offered by brand-name thyroid hormone replacement pills. Common dosages for thyroid cancer patients on levothyroxine sodium are 125 or 137. The appropriate range for TSH suppression is anywhere from 100 to 200 micrograms; for example, in my own case, my TSH suppression dosage is 150 micrograms.

One study found that patients on thyroid hormone specifically for TSH suppression were better off waiting one hour after taking their pill in the morning before having breakfast. It was suspected that milk products had something to do with improving the absorption of the medication.

If You're Elderly or Have Heart Disease

To avoid any risk of being "overreplaced" (overdosed to the point where you're hyperthyroid), dosages of thyroid hormone in your case should start fairly low, at around 12.5 micrograms (a 25-microgram pill cut in half with a special pill cutter, available at all pharmacies). Dosages should be adjusted very, very slowly, in increments of 25 micrograms until you reach the right thyroid level.

What Brand Should I Take?

The key phrase in a quality thyroid hormone replacement pill is "precise dosing." This enables your doctor to prescribe the lowest, most effective dose without overdoing it, or "underdoing" it. It's also important to keep in mind that thyroid hormone brands are not interchangeable. Endocrinologists have seen as much as a four-fold difference in thyroid function after patients have switched brands. The right dose for you on Brand A may not be the right dose for you on Brand B.

That said, studies done to date show no significant differences between the four most commonly dispensed brands of levothyroxine sodium. In ClinicalSpeak, they were found to be "bioequivalent" (absorbed in the blood in precisely the same way) and were considered bioequivalent under the current guidelines of the Food and Drug Administration criteria. That means the brands studied were found to be interchangeable in the majority of patients receiving thyroid hormone replacement therapy. But there is disagreement about bioequivalency amongst thyroid brands.

For instance, one manufacturer had to recall some of its batches from the market because the batches were made from "nonmicronized" raw materials from another supplier, which meant that the drug was not being made available to the body appropriately (called bioavailability). Very simple changes in the manufacturing of levothyroxine tablets can make a big difference in the performance of the tablets. In addition, when the batch of thyroid pills that you receive from your pharmacist has been hanging around on the shelf for too long, the pills may not be as potent as they were when first shipped. Therefore, it's crucial to always ask when your pills *expire*. Experts also warn that a bottle of pills that expires in March 2002 that is dispensed in December 2001 should be rejected by the buyer as a batch that is not "fresh."

The shortest route to maintaining thyroid hormone function with your thyroid pill is to:

1. Choose a brand of thyroid hormone pill that offers *precise dosing* (see Table 3.1). This is particularly important for women over forty, who may be approaching menopause, anyone over sixty, and people with heart conditions.

2. If you feel good, stay on that brand. Since you may require a different dose on Brand A than you do on Brand B, just stay on the brand you're on. If you don't feel balanced, you'll need to investigate other brands.

3. Watch for signs of hyperthyroidism (see Table 3.2). These symptoms mean that you're on too high a dosage of thyroid hormone.

4. Watch for signs of hypothyroidism (see Chapter 1). These are signs that you're on too low a dosage of thyroid hormone, or possibly the wrong brand.

5. Get a thyroid function test every three months for the first couple of years after you begin your pills; then graduate to six months; then annually.

6. Always find out when the pills dispensed expire, and how long they've been on the pharmacist's shelf.

7. If you miss a pill, don't worry about it, just carry on the next day. Thyroid hormone pills have a very long half-life and missing a pill every now and then won't make any difference. If you accidentally take two pills, again, this won't make any difference. Just carry on.

8. Take your pill on an empty stomach if you can. Don't take it at the same time as your multivitamin; wait at least two hours after taking your pill before you add the multivitamin.

The Synthroid Scandal

The reason we know that there is no difference in bioequivalency between thyroid hormone brands is because Knoll Pharmaceutical, makers of Synthroid, initiated and funded the research that showed this. A scandal arose when Knoll decided not to publish the results of this research for seven years. In April 1997, the *Journal of the American Medical Association* published the research results anyway, while Knoll insisted that the results were kept from the public because the research was flawed, and the results invalid.

In May 1997, a class action suit was filed against Knoll, claiming that thyroid patients overpaid in that seven-year time span for Synthroid by as much as three times the price of competitors' products. The lawsuit demanded that patients be compensated by Knoll for their overpayment.

A settlement has been reached in the Synthroid Marketing Litigation (Case No. 97 C 6017, MDL No. 1182, in the United States District Court for the Northern District of Illinois). The proposed settlement fund comes to $87.4 million for consumers who purchased Synthroid between January 1, 1990, and October 21, 1999, and claimants had until March 10, 2000, to file their claims. As long as you live in the United States or Puerto Rico and purchased Synthroid within these time frames, and filed your claim in time (there were many ads in national magazines about this), you were eligible to receive money from this settlement fund. Don't get too upset if you missed the deadline, though. For example, if 800,000 people file a claim as a "pre-1995" purchaser, each person will get $119. Not a great loss! For more information about this class action suit, call 1-800-853-4853 or go to the Web site: www.synthroidclaims.com. You can also write to: Synthroid Marketing Litigation, P.O. Box 7090, San Rafael, CA 94912-7090.

What's In This Stuff, Anyway?

Thyroid hormone pills contain a number of excipients (substances added to a medicine, which allow it to be formed into a shape and consistency). These include lubricants, binders, and disintegrants. The pills may contain acacia, lactose, magnesium stearate, povidone, confectioner's sugar (which has cornstarch), and talc. The lactose used in thyroid hormone pills is minimal; there is approximately one hundred times the amount of lactose in one-half cup of whole milk as in one tablet of Synthroid, for example. If you're highly lactose intolerant, you can take your thyroid hormone pill together with a lactase enzyme.

When You Need T3

As you may recall from Chapter 1, there are two thyroid hormones produced by the thyroid gland—thyroxine, known as T4 (four iodine atoms), and triiodothyronine, known as T3 (three iodine atoms). (See page 2).

Over the years, many of my readers have written to me about just not "feeling right" on their thyroid hormone pills, even though their TSH levels were normal, and they were apparently on the right dosage. An article published in the February 11, 1999, issue of the *New England Journal of Medicine* reported on some dramatic findings for thyroid patients. Apparently, when the thyroid hormone with three iodine atoms (T3), known as triiodothyronine, was added to their regular thyroid hormone replacement pill (which is thyroxine, or T4, the thyroid hormone with four iodine atoms), people felt much better. A cocktail of T3 and T4 helped relieve depression, brain fog, fatigue, and other hypothyroid symptoms (see Chapter 2). In this study, thirty-three patients with severe hypothyroidism were treated alternatively with pure thyroxine (T4) or a lower dose of T4 plus triiodothyronine (T3). The article concluded that "treatment with thyroxine plus triiodothyronine improved the quality of life for most [hypothyroid] patients."

This may explain why some patients have felt better on alternative thyroid drugs such as the natural Armour Thyroid, Westhroid, and Naturethroid, which contain T4 and T3 naturally, and the synthetic T4/T3 drug Thyrolar. T3 can also be added to your regular thyroid hormone pill as an additional pill, known as Cytomel®, which is simply pure T3, or triiodothyronine.

This comes as surprising and welcome news for many thyroid patients who thought they were suffering from phantom hypothyroid symptoms. A survey conducted by The Thyroid Foundation of America found that 59 percent of survey participants complained of persisting hypothyroid symptoms, such as muscle aches, lethargy, and/or depression. As a result, T3 is now a common addition to T4 for many hypothyroid patients.

If you're currently not feeling quite right on your thyroid hormone pill, get a copy of the article and bring it to your doctor's attention. Or photocopy this page and bring it into your doctor's office! Then sit down and have a frank discussion about whether you stand to benefit from T3 therapy.

Risks of T3 Therapy

The problem with T3 therapy is that many thyroid patients look upon it as a "miracle cure." They ascribe all kinds of benefits to this therapy that may not be there for them, especially if they have other health problems, such as heart disease, high blood pressure, high cholesterol, and so on.

T3 therapy can benefit some people, but harm others—particularly elderly patients with other health problems. For example, T3 therapy is not recommended for people with angina, and it can also cause you to become hyperthyroid, meaning that you may suffer from chest pain, increased pulse rate, palpitations, excessive sweating, heat intolerance, nervousness, and other hyperthyroid symptoms. It is also not recommended for people taking imipramine and other tricyclic antidepressants.

Like many new therapies, T3 therapy has not been tested on groups of people who in the past were abused in medical research: elderly people, minority groups, and women. For example, studies that looked at heart disease excluded women, and now we're seeing that heart disease manifests differently in women than in men. As a result of medical ignorance surrounding women's heart disease, many women have needlessly died, sent home with their heart attack symptoms. Therefore, serious questions remain about whether T3 works differently in men than in women, particularly postmenopausal women, whose risk of heart disease increases because of estrogen loss. The published study using T3 therapy was conducted on a small sample of thyroid patients (thirty-three), with an average age of forty-six, who were taking T3 therapy for only ten weeks. So, what we don't know about T3 therapy are answers to the following questions:

1. What are the long-term effects of T3 therapy?
2. How does T3 affect people sixty-five years and older?
3. How does T3 affect women past menopause who are not taking hormone replacement therapy?
4. How does T3 affect women past menopause who *are* taking hormone replacement therapy?
5. How does T3 affect children?
6. How does T3 affect pregnant women or women who are breast-feeding?
7. How does T3 affect people of different races and ethnic backgrounds?
8. How does T3 therapy affect people with other health problems, such as heart disease or diabetes, or people who have undergone cancer therapy?
9. How does T3 therapy interact with other drugs, including antidepressants, blood thinners, nonsteroidal anti-inflammatory drugs (NSAIDs), and so on?

Because T3 is so potent, it must be administered only if you're being closely monitored. That doesn't mean you can't take advantage of this therapy if you feel you have something to gain; it simply means that you must be informed of the unknown risks before you go on this treatment.

Thyroid Replacement Hormone and Other Drugs

Because we all either combine various medications from time to time, or are taking other daily medications for different health conditions, it's important to be aware of how thyroid replacement hormone medication interacts with other prescription and nonprescription drugs.

Oral Anticoagulants (Coumadin, Warfarin, Heparin)

An anticoagulant, or blood thinner, helps prevent blood clotting and *is not as useful for preventing heart attacks as it is for preventing strokes. This drug dissolves clots.* When combined with thyroid hormone, the anticoagulant can become more potent, which could cause some minor hemorrhaging. Your doctor may need to reduce the dosage of your anticoagulant. This occurs only when initiating thyroxine therapy, not when patients are taking it chronically. When an elderly patient is on these drugs, his or her thyroid levels should be tested every six months.

Estrogen

This combination can increase your T4 (thyroxine) readings. It's best to get your thyroid levels checked once a year if you're taking estrogen for any reason.

Insulin or Oral Hypoglycemics

This combination lowers the effect of insulin, which means that your doctor may have to increase your insulin dosage. This occurs only when you begin to take thyroid hormone tablets. After both medications are adjusted, you should be fine. If you're diabetic, however, it's a good idea to get your thyroid levels checked once a year.

Anticonvulsants

Drugs such as Dilantin are prescribed for epilepsy. They help to prevent seizures. This combination lowers your T4 levels. This doesn't

mean that you'll automatically become hypothyroid, but you'll probably need a lower dose and should have your thyroid levels checked
about once a year.

Laxatives, Coffee, or Alcohol

Thyroxine and anything that affects the digestive system should be
taken as many hours apart as possible to ensure better absorption of
the thyroid medication.

Cholestyramine

This drug is prescribed for people who have high cholesterol levels.
When combined with thyroxine, this drug lowers the absorption of
thyroxine. Therefore, the two should not be taken together. A space
of three to four hours between each is recommended, with thyroxine
being taken first.

Antidepressants

If you're on thyroid replacement hormone and are taking any one of
the following antidepressant drugs, the antidepressant drug will
become more potent: Elavil, Ascendin, Etrofon, Limbitral, Pamelor,
Surmontil, Tofranil, Tofranil P.M., Triavil, or Norpramin. This can also
lead to abnormal heart rhythms. This only happens when you first
begin your thyroid medication, however, and tapers off when your
medications are balanced. Make sure that you get your thyroid levels
checked every year, and that you inform whoever is managing your
antidepressant medication that you are taking thyroid hormone.

Lithium

Lithium is prescribed for bipolar disorder (formerly known as manic
depression). Even if your thyroid is functioning normally, lithium can
cause hypothyroidism; roughly 8 to 11 percent of people on lithium
do become hypothyroid. Lithium has also been known to cause goiter
and hyperthyroidism, and to trigger Graves' disease. Insist that your

thyroid levels be checked every six months while you're on lithium. In between, you might want to keep a log of your moods on a day-to-day basis. If you're feeling unusually depressed for long periods of time, get your thyroid levels checked, just in case.

Amiodarone

This is a drug used to treat atrial fibrillation, a heart rhythm problem. This drug contains a lot of iodine, and it's been found to induce both hypo- and hyperthyroidism, but in North America, where we have sufficient iodine, hypothyroidism is more common. It's also been found to accelerate Hashimoto's disease, but does not cause it in people who do not suffer from it initially. Hyperthyroidism is caused by this drug if you have a toxic multinodular goiter. If you're vulnerable to thyroid disease and you're on this drug, request an antithyroid antibody test just in case. Since the drug is stored in body fat, it can induce a thyroid problem up to twelve months after it's been stopped.

Corticosteroids

These can suppress TSH and interfere with thyroid hormone production in the body.

Certain Anesthetics

Ketamine, a type of anesthetic, can cause your heart to race if you're on synthetic thyroid hormone.

4

The Hypothyroid Diet

I'VE CULLED ALL the information I have on diet and nutrition (and it's a lot!) to create what I call "The Hypothyroid Diet." Since everything slows down when you're hypothyroid, you need to know how to eat and what to eat in order to compensate for your body's slowness during this time, as well as how to avoid complications of hypothyroidism. The right diet can help improve constipation and bloat, fatigue, and weight gain. In essence, this is a diet that will help you feel better while combating periods of hypothyroidism when you're not properly balanced on medication, while also helping to prevent cardiovascular and colon health problems. It will also complement your thyroid medication, if you are balanced right now. And finally, it will help you combat a preexisting weight problem (see Chapter 2), which may be aggravated by your hypothyroidism.

Battling the Bloat

Feeling bloated and constipated is a classic hypothyroid ailment. Much of the bloat is actually caused by constipation, and also by not drinking enough water. Few people understand that when you increase fiber, you have to increase water intake. Here's what you need to know about fiber and water.

Understanding Fiber

Fiber is the part of a plant your body can't digest. It comes in the form of both water-soluble fiber (which dissolves in water) and water-insoluble fiber (which does not dissolve in water but instead absorbs water); this is what's meant by "soluble" and "insoluble" fiber. Soluble and insoluble fiber do differ, but they are equally beneficial.

Soluble fiber, somehow, lowers the "bad" cholesterol, or low-density lipids (LDL), in your body. Experts aren't entirely sure how soluble fiber works its magic, but one popular theory is that it gets mixed into the bile the liver secretes, and forms a type of gel that traps the building blocks of cholesterol, thus lowering your LDL levels. It's akin to a spider web trapping smaller insects.

Insoluble fiber doesn't affect your cholesterol levels at all, but it regulates your bowel movements. How does it do this? As the insoluble fiber moves through your digestive tract, it absorbs water like a sponge and helps to form your waste into a solid form faster, making the stools larger, softer, and easier to pass. Without insoluble fiber, your solid waste just gets pushed down to the colon or lower intestine as always, where it is stored and dried out until you're ready to have a bowel movement. High-starch foods are associated with drier stools. This is exacerbated when you "ignore the urge," as the colon will dehydrate the waste even more until it becomes harder and more difficult to pass, a condition known as constipation. Insoluble fiber will help to regulate your bowel movements by speeding things along. Insoluble fiber increases the "transit time" by increasing colon motility and limiting the time dietary toxins "hang around" the intestinal wall. This is why it can dramatically decrease your risk of colon cancer.

Good sources of soluble fiber include oats or oat bran, legumes (dried beans and peas), some seeds, carrots, oranges, bananas, and other fruits. Soybeans are also high sources of soluble fiber. Studies show that people with very high cholesterol have the most to gain by eating soybeans. Soybean is also a *phytoestrogen* (plant estrogen) that is believed to lower the risk of estrogen-related cancers (for example, breast cancer), as well as lower the incidence of estrogen-loss symptoms associated with menopause.

Good sources of insoluble fiber are wheat bran and whole grains, skins from various fruits and vegetables, seeds, leafy greens, and cruciferous vegetables (cauliflower, broccoli, and brussels sprouts). The problem is understanding what is truly "whole grain." For example, there is an assumption that because bread is dark or brown, it's more nutritious; this isn't so. In fact, many brown breads are simply enriched white breads dyed with molasses. ("Enriched" means that nutrients lost during processing have been replaced.) High-fiber pita breads and bagels are available, but you have to search for them. A good rule is to simply look for the phrase "whole wheat," which means that the wheat is, indeed, whole.

What's in a Grain?

Most of us will turn to grains and cereals to boost our fiber intake, which experts recommend should be at about 25 to 35 grams per day. Use this to help gauge whether you're getting enough. The following list measures the amount of insoluble fiber in various cereals and breads. If you're a little under "par," an easy way to boost your fiber intake is to simply add pure wheat bran to your foods, available in health food stores or supermarkets in a sort of "sawdust" format. Three tablespoons of wheat bran is equal to 4.4 grams of fiber. Sprinkle 1 to 2 tablespoons onto cereals, rice, pasta, or meat dishes. You can also sprinkle it into orange juice or lowfat yogurt. It has virtually no calories, but it's important to drink a glass of water with your wheat bran, as well as a glass of water after you've finished your wheat bran-enriched meal.

Keep in mind that some of the newer high-fiber breads on the market today have up to 7 grams of fiber per slice. This chart is based on what is normally found in typical grocery stores.

Cereals	Grams of Fiber
(based on 1 cup unless otherwise specified)	
Fiber First	15.0
Fiber One	12.8
All Bran	10.0
Oatmeal	5.0
Raisin Bran (¾ cup)	4.6
Bran Flakes	4.4
Shreddies (⅔ cup)	2.7
Cheerios	2.2
Corn Flakes (1½ cups)	0.8
Special K (1½ cups)	0.4
Rice Krispies (1½ cups)	0.3

Breads	Grams of Fiber
(based on 1 slice)	
Rye	2.0
Pumpernickel	2.0
12-grain	1.7
100 percent whole wheat	1.3
Raisin	1.0
Cracked wheat	1.0
White	0

Fruits and Veggies

Another easy way of boosting fiber content is to know how much fiber your fruits and vegetables pack per serving. All fruits, beans (aka legumes), and vegetables listed here show measurements for insoluble fiber, which is not only good for colon health, but for your heart. Some of these numbers may surprise you!

Fruit	Grams of Fiber
Raspberries (¾ cup)	6.4
Strawberries (1 cup)	4.0
Blackberries (½ cup)	3.9

Orange (1)	3.0
Apple (1)	2.0
Pear (½ medium)	2.0
Grapefruit (½ cup)	1.1
Kiwi (1)	1.0

Beans	Grams of Fiber

(based on ½ cup unless otherwise specified)

Green beans	4.0
White beans	3.6
Kidney beans	3.3
Pinto beans	3.3
Lima beans	3.2

Vegetables	Grams of Fiber

(based on ½ cup unless otherwise specified)

Potato, baked with skin (1 large)	4.0
Acorn squash	3.8
Peas	3.0
Corn, creamed, canned	2.7
Brussels sprouts	2.3
Asparagus (¾ cup)	2.3
Corn kernels	2.1
Zucchini	1.4
Carrots (cooked)	1.2
Broccoli	1.1

Drinking Water with Fiber

How many people do you know who say, ". . . But I *do* eat tons of fiber and I'm still constipated!"? Probably quite a few. Well, the reason they remain constipated in spite of their high-fiber diet is because they are not drinking *water* with their fiber. Water means water. Milk, coffee, tea, sodas, or juice are not a substitute for water. Unless you drink water with your fiber, the fiber will not "bulk up" in your colon to create the nice, soft bowel movements you so desire. Think of fiber as a sponge. Obviously, a dry sponge won't work. You must soak it with water in order for it to be useful. Same thing here. Fiber without water is as useful as a dry sponge. *You gotta soak your fiber!* Here is the fiber/water recipe:

- Drink two glasses of water with your fiber. This means having a glass of water with whatever you're eating. Even if what you're eating does not contain much fiber, drinking water with your meal is a good habit to get into!
- Drink two glasses of water after you eat.

There are, of course, other reasons to drink lots of water throughout the day. For example, some studies show that dehydration can lead to mood swings and depression. Women are often advised from numerous health and beauty experts to drink eight to ten glasses of water per day for other reasons: water helps you to lose weight, have well-hydrated, beautiful skin, and urinate regularly, which is important for bladder form and function (women, in particular, can suffer from bladder infections and urinary incontinence). By drinking water with your fiber, you'll be able to get up to that "eight glasses of water per day" in no time.

Understanding Constipation

Before you can deal with constipation, it's important to understand what constitutes normal bowel habits. The colon essentially acts as a solid waste container, drying out the waste that doesn't get absorbed further up. The nervous system controls the muscular contractions of the colon, which slowly move the waste downward, toward the rectum. We experience these stronger muscular contractions as "the urge." Once we feel the urge, we sit down, relax, and allow the gentle contractions to overtake us. All we have to do is relax and the anal sphincter will open to allow the passage of stool.

The frequency of bowel movements varies from person to person. Although many North American sources say it's "normal" to move your bowels anywhere from a few times per day to a few times per week, if you're not having one to three large, bulky, soft but firm bowel movements per day, you probably have a tendency to be constipated. A normal stool is solid or "formed" but not hard, and certainly should not contain mucus or blood. The stools should pass without cramps, pain, or strain. However, normal stools can pass noisily, since natural gas (called flatus)—swallowed air (nitrogen) that gets trapped in the lower intestine—often comes out with the stools, or independently.

Constipation means that you are not experiencing an urge to move your bowels, and when you do, the stools are hard and difficult to pass. Generally, if more than three days have passed since your last bowel movement, the stools will harden. The colon will continue to dry out the stools because that's what the colon does.

In the absence of a condition such as hypothyroidism, most constipation is "functional" in that there is no disease or organic problem at work; it's a lifestyle problem, having to do with ignoring the urge to go (if you're surrounded by public toilets, for example), or not allowing enough time in the morning to *create* the urge to go by drinking or eating something. If you ignore the urge too often, you may stop feeling an urge altogether. Studies comparing bowel habits of North Americans to Africans show that the incidence of colon cancer is higher in North Americans, who have less frequent bowel movements than do Africans. We can learn from these studies and modify our lifestyles accordingly. The idea is to find a happy medium, because chronic diarrhea is also dangerous to your health. In fact, it's far more troublesome than chronic constipation.

If your constipation is a more sudden or recent occurrence in your life, then there could be other causes in addition to hypothyroidism, such as:

- Pregnancy or changes in the menstrual cycle. It's not unusual for women to experience constipation at these times.
- Hot weather. When you're perspiring and losing body fluid, you could become constipated.
- Stress.
- Travel (changes in schedule, diet, and time zones can interfere with regularity).
- Anal sores (this includes fissures, hemorrhoids, or herpes).

- Medications (particularly pain control medications in chronic illness).
- Periods of vomiting and diarrhea.

Chronic Constipation

Chronic constipation can be caused by a variety of things, including laxative abuse, diseases affecting body tissues and nerve or muscle control, inflammation, scarring or blockage in the lower intestine, spinal injuries, and prolonged bedrest or being bedridden (especially seniors). But again, lack of exercise and poor diet are the most common causes of chronic constipation.

Staying Regular Without Laxatives

If you're not moving your bowels at least once a day, you can probably change this by modifying your diet or lifestyle. Most often, *not* eating enough soluble fiber, *not* drinking enough water, and *not* getting enough exercise are the causes of constipation. Exercise helps to strengthen your abdominal muscles, and helps blood and oxygen circulate throughout your body—which simply makes *everything* work better. (See the next chapter for more details.)

The best way to know the "right" laxatives is to know the *wrong* ones. What you want to avoid is anything that is a *stimulant laxative*, which can include "herbal" laxatives, such as senna and cascara sagrada. There is some contradictory information regarding cascara sagrada, however. Many herbalists maintain that cascara sagrada, unlike senna, is considered more of a "tonic" than a laxative, and is said not to create a dependency, and in fact, may be helpful for your colon. However, like other stimulant laxatives, it works by stimulating the colon to contract, creating a bowel movement and, with too much use, a dependency. The medical advisor for this book strongly advises against using cascara sagrada. A dependency on laxatives means that you will not be able to move your bowels without the laxative because your colon becomes "used" to it.

There are several herbal teas and herbal concoctions that promote digestion and regularity through harmless spices or ingredients. You may have heard of acidophilus (liquid or powder) as a remedy for chronic constipation, which does not create a dependency. Or, in Ayurvedic medicine (an ancient Indian healing system), *triphala* is taken to promote regularity and good digestion. Triphala is a combination of three ancient Ayurvedic ingredients: haritaki, bibhitaki, and amalaki. It can be found in most health food stores. In addition, the following spices are good for digestion, and are not harmful to your colon in any way: licorice root, peppermint leaf, anise seed, yellow dock root, dandelion root, rose petals, coriander seed, celery seed, cinnamon bark, ginger root, cardamom seed, clove bud, and black pepper.

If you must have an occasional laxative, the best kind are bulking agents, which are sold as laxatives, but are not laxatives per se. Metamucil is an example of a bulking agent. Adopting a "water with fiber routine" will probably cure you of constipation. Try that first before you try a laxative. If nothing is working, and you haven't moved your bowels in five or six days, try inserting a glycerin suppository overnight and in the morning, which should get things moving. If there's still no action, the next step is to try an enema, and after that, a mild laxative, such as milk of magnesia. Finally, you may have a bowel obstruction of some sort, which a good gastroenterologist can discover.

By simply obeying your urges, you can avoid constipation. Learning to suppress the urge to defecate can create what is called a "lazy bowel." When you feel the urge to defecate, drop what you're doing and get to the toilet. We all know ways of excusing ourselves to make or take "important calls." Why not make your nature call the most important call of your day?

Another way to obey the nature call is to give yourself enough time to receive the call in the first place. If you get out of bed and rush out the door immediately, you may be one of millions who suffers from "commuter constipation."

For many, years of ignoring our urges and laxative dependency has made it impossible to "go it alone." Take heart: You can retrain your bowel to recapture its youth. Here's the recipe:

- Drink a glass of warm water in the morning as soon as you get up, and insert a glycerin suppository into your rectum.
- Move around a bit (make your bed, do some stretches) for three or four minutes.

- Sit on the toilet and gently push for about two minutes. If nothing happens, get up and leave.

If you practice this routine every day for three to six months, you should be able to retrain your colon to have a bowel movement when you drink warm water in the morning. In other words, the warm water will stimulate your colon. Missing even a day of this routine could set you back weeks, though!

A Word About Hemorrhoids

The straining caused by chronic constipation can lead to hemorrhoids. These are swollen blood vessels or veins around the anus or inside (internal) covered by the inner lining. A classic symptom of internal hemorrhoids is finding bright red blood squirting into the toilet water, covering your stool, on toilet paper, or in the toilet bowl. Sometimes an internal hemorrhoid is large enough that it protrudes through your rectum, and hangs outside the body, known as a *protruding hemorrhoid*. Since bleeding is a problem with internal hemorrhoids, you can become anemic.

To find some relief, try warm tub or sitz baths (when the water just covers your "hiny") several times a day. Don't use anything in the water except a little baking soda (optional), and don't stay in longer than about ten minutes. Stool softeners may help you pass stool more comfortably, while ice packs will help reduce swelling (ten minutes on/ten minutes off). Frequently shifting your position while standing or sitting is helpful. Over-the-counter medication such as Preparation H can also give you relief but won't shrink the hemorrhoid. If the problem is not resolving itself, the hemorrhoid can be removed in your doctor's office.

Improving Digestion

Hypothyroidism can interfere with normal digestion and absorption of nutrients. The following spices can aid digestion:

- *Coriander.* Eases gases and works to tone the digestive system. Use powdered or whole seed, or garnish with fresh leaves (cilantro).

- *Cardamom.* Reduces the mucus-forming effects of dairy products. Use powdered or whole seeds.
- *Turmeric.* Generally improves metabolism and helps you to digest proteins. Use the root ground. (Gives dishes a yellowish color and can stain clothes and china.)
- *Black pepper.* Stimulates appetite and helps you digest dairy products. Use freshly ground.
- *Cumin.* Helps reduce gases and generally tones the digestive system. Use seeds whole or powdered.
- *Fennel.* Helps prevent gas. Chew the seeds after eating, or add them to vegetables that tend to produce gas when cooking. Use whole or powdered.
- *Ginger.* This aids digestion and respiration. Also helps to relieve gas and constipation, or indigestion. Use root fresh or dried. (Note: Ginger can aggravate bleeding ulcers, however.)
- *Cinnamon.* This naturally cleanses your digestive system. Use powdered, in sticks or pieces.
- *Nutmeg.* This helps your body absorb nutrients from food, but should be used sparingly.
- *Clove.* This helps your body absorb nutrients. Use whole or ground.
- *Cayenne.* This helps to stimulate your digestive juices, and is known for having a "cleansing action" within the large intestine. Helps to relieve that feeling of "fullness" after eating a heavy meal.
- *Licorice root.* Take two to four capsules after meals as a general digestive aid.

Cut Out Caffeine

Caffeine is hard on the gut. By cutting it down or out, many people find that their digestion improves. Here's a checklist of how much caffeine some foods contain, with the milligrams of caffeine given.

Coffee (5-ounce cup)	Milligrams
Brewed, drip method	60–180
Brewed, percolator	40–170

Instant	30–120
Decaffeinated, brewed	2–5
Decaffeinated, instant	1–5

Tea (5-ounce cup)	Milligrams
Brewed, major brands	20–90
Brewed, imported brands	25–110
Instant	25–50
Iced, 12-ounce glass	67–76

Other	Milligrams
6-ounce glass of caffeine-containing soda	15–30
5-ounce cup of cocoa beverage	2–20
8-ounce glass of chocolate milk	2–7
1-ounce unce serving of milk chocolate	1–15
1-ounce serving of dark chocolate, semi-sweet	5–35
Single square of Baker's chocolate	26
Serving of chocolate-flavored syrup	4

Quit Smoking

Smoking can aggravate all kinds of thyroid problems, particularly thyroid eye disease (see *The Thyroid Sourcebook, 4th edition*). Smoking is also, of course, hard on the lungs and heart. But did you know that it's also hard on the gut? If you're having digestion problems that are aggravated by hypothyroidism, by quitting smoking you may be able to make your symptoms vanish.

Enjoy a good cigar or a pipe once in a while? Forget it—cigars are bad for the gut, too. When you smoke a cigar, you're getting filler, binder, and wrapper, which are made of air-cured and fermented tobaccos. Like cigarette tobacco, lit cigars emit over four thousand chemicals, of which forty-three are known to cause cancer—many of them gastrointestinal cancers.

Cigar smokers have higher death rates than nonsmokers for most smoking-related diseases, although they are not nearly as high as for cigarette smokers. When the nicotine is absorbed through the mouth, however, cigar/pipe smokers, as well as anyone using chewing tobacco or snuff, are at higher risk of laryngeal, oral, and esophageal cancer. Cigar/pipe smokers also have higher death rates than nonsmokers from chronic obstructive lung disease as well as lung cancer.

Whether it's cigars, cigarettes, or even chewing tobacco (snuff), take a look at some of the things you'll gain by quitting smoking:

- improved digestion and a sense of taste
- decreased risk of heart disease
- decreased risk of cancer (includes lung, esophagus, mouth, throat, pancreas, kidney, bladder, and cervix)
- lower heart rate and blood pressure
- decreased risk of lung disease (bronchitis, emphysema)
- relaxation of blood vessels
- better teeth
- fewer wrinkles

Not everyone can quit smoking "cold turkey," although it's a strategy that many have used successfully. (Some "cold turkey" quitters report that keeping one package of cigarettes within reach lessens anxiety.) The symptoms of nicotine withdrawal begin within a few hours and peak at twenty-four to forty-eight hours after quitting. You may experience anxiety, irritability, hostility, restlessness, insomnia, and anger. For these reasons, many smokers turn to smoking cessation programs, which can include some of the following:

• *Herbal and homeopathic smoking cessation aids.* There are many herbal and homeopathic smoking cessation products available. Some use plant sources to reduce cravings; some work by using natural substances to help you "detox." Contact your local natural pharmacy or health/herbal retailer for more information.

• *Behavioral counseling.* Behavioral counseling, either group or individual, can raise the rate of abstinence to 20 to 25 percent. This approach to smoking cessation aims to change the mental processes of smoking, reinforce the benefits of nonsmoking, and teach skills to help the smoker avoid the urge to smoke.

- *Nicotine gum.* Nicotine (Nicorette) gum is now available over the counter. It works as an aid to help you quit smoking by reducing nicotine cravings and withdrawal symptoms. Nicotine gum helps you wean yourself from nicotine by allowing you to gradually decrease the dosage until you stop using it altogether, a process that usually takes about twelve weeks. The only disadvantage with this method is that it caters to the oral and addictive aspects of smoking (rewarding the "urge" to smoke with a dose of nicotine).

- *Nicotine patch.* Transdermal nicotine, or the "patch" (Habitrol, Nicoderm, Nicotrol), doubles abstinence rates in former smokers. Most brands are now available over the counter. Each morning, a new patch is applied to a different area of dry, clean, hairless skin and left on for the day. Some patches are designed to be worn a full twenty-four hours. However, the constant supply of nicotine to the bloodstream sometimes causes very vivid or disturbing dreams. You can also expect to feel a mild itching, burning, or tingling at the site of the patch when it is first applied. The nicotine patch works best when it is worn for at least seven to twelve weeks, with a gradual decrease in strength (i.e., nicotine). Many smokers find it effective because it allows them to tackle the psychological addiction to smoking before they are forced to deal with the physical symptoms of withdrawal.

- *Nicotine inhaler.* The nicotine inhaler (Nicotrol Inhaler) delivers nicotine orally via inhalation from a plastic tube. Its success rate is about 28 percent, similar to that of nicotine gum. It's available by prescription only in the United States, and has yet to make its debut in Canada. Like nicotine gum, the inhaler mimics smoking behavior by responding to each craving or "urge" to smoke, a feature that has both advantages and disadvantages to the smoker who wants to get over the physical symptoms of withdrawal. The nicotine inhaler should be used for a period of twelve weeks.

- *Nicotine nasal spray.* Like nicotine gum and the nicotine patch, the nasal spray reduces cravings and withdrawal symptoms, allowing smokers to cut back gradually. One squirt delivers about 1 milligram of nicotine. In three clinical trials involving 730 patients, 31 to 35 percent were not smoking at six months. This compares to an average of 12 to 15 percent of smokers who were able to quit unaided. The nasal spray has a couple of advantages over the gum and the patch: Nicotine is rapidly absorbed across the nasal membranes, providing a kick that is more like the real thing; and the prompt onset of action plus a flexible dosing schedule benefits heavier smokers. Because the nicotine reaches your bloodstream so quickly, nasal sprays do have a greater potential for addiction than the slower-acting gum and patch. Nasal sprays are not yet available for use in Canada.

• *Alternative therapies.* Hypnosis, meditation, and acupuncture have helped some smokers quit. In the cases of hypnosis and meditation, sessions may be private or part of a group smoking cessation program.

Drugs That Help You Quit

The drug bupropion (Zyban) is now available and is an option for people who have been unsuccessful using nicotine replacement. Formerly prescribed as an antidepressant, bupropion was "discovered" by accident: Researchers knew that quitting smokers were often depressed and so they began experimenting with the drug as a means to fight depression, not addiction. Bupropion reduces the withdrawal symptoms associated with smoking cessation and can be used in conjunction with nicotine replacement therapy. Researchers suspect that bupropion works directly in the brain to disrupt the addictive power of nicotine by affecting the same chemical neurotransmitters (or "messengers") in the brain, such as dopamine, that nicotine does.

The pleasurable aspect of addictive drugs such as nicotine and cocaine is triggered by the release of dopamine. Smoking floods the brain with dopamine. *The New England Journal of Medicine* published the results of a study of more than six hundred smokers taking bupropion. At the end of treatment, 44 percent of those who took the highest dose of the drug (300 milligrams) were not smoking, compared to 19 percent of the group who took a placebo. By the end of one year, 23 percent of the 300-milligram group and 12 percent of the placebo group were still smoke-free. Using Zyban *with* nicotine replacement therapy seems to improve the quit rate a bit further. Four-week quit rates from the study were 23 percent for placebo, 36 percent for the patch; 49 percent for Zyban, and 58 percent for the combination of Zyban and the patch.

Battling Fatigue

Fatigue, brain fog, lethargy, and depression can be improved with the right diet, too. We now know there are a variety of daily nutrients that help to regulate our energy levels and moods. Tryptophan, for example, which is found in milk and other dairy products, helps our bodies to build neurotransmitters, such as serotonin.

The B vitamins are also important for our mental health. Vitamin B_{12} is crucial for good general health, while other B-complex vitamins (thiamine, riboflavin, niacin, pyridoxine, pantothenic acid, and biotin) are essential for brain function, enabling you to be cognizant and alert. You'll find the B vitamins in lean meats, whole grains, liver, seeds, nuts, wheat germ, and dairy products. Folate (aka folic acid) is particularly important for a healthy mood. It is found in liver, eggs, leafy greens, yeast, legumes, whole grains, nuts, fruits (bananas, orange juice, grapefruit juice), and vegetables (broccoli, spinach, asparagus, brussels sprouts). When you don't have enough "brain foods" you can become more prone to stress, anxiety, or depression.

Calcium and magnesium aid your brain to properly transmit nerve impulses. Calcium is found in dairy products, leafy greens, eggs, and fish (particularly salmon and sardines); soy, nuts, whole grains, milk, meat, and fish contain magnesium. The following tells you where to find various nutrients from natural sources.

- *Vitamin A/beta carotene.* Found in liver, fish oils, egg yolk, whole milk, butter; beta carotene—leafy greens, yellow and orange vegetables and fruits. Depleted by coffee, alcohol, cortisone, mineral oil, fluorescent lights, liver "cleansing," excessive intake of iron, or a lack of protein.

- *Vitamin B_6.* Found in meats, poultry, fish, nuts, liver, bananas, avocados, grapes, pears, egg yolk, whole grains, and legumes.

- *Vitamin B_{12}.* Found in meats, dairy products, eggs, liver, fish. Both B_{12} and B_6 are depleted by coffee, alcohol, tobacco, sugar, raw oysters, and birth control pills.

- *Vitamin C.* Found in citrus fruits, broccoli, green peppers, strawberries, cabbage, tomatos, cantaloupes, potatoes, leafy greens. Herbal sources: rose hips, yellow dock root, raspberry leaves, red clover, hops, nettles, pine needles, dandelion greens, alfalfa, echinacea, skullcap, parsley, cayenne, and paprika. Depleted by antibiotics, aspirin and other pain relievers, coffee, stress, aging, smoking, baking soda, and high fever.

• *Vitamin D.* Found in fortified milk, butter, leafy green vegetables, egg yolk, fish oils, liver, skin exposure to sunlight, shrimp. Herbal sources: none; not found in plants. Depleted by mineral oil used on the skin, frequent baths, sunscreens with SPF 8 or higher.

• *Vitamin E.* Found in nuts, seeds, whole grains, fish-liver oils, freshly leafy greens, kale, cabbage, asparagus. Herbal sources: alfalfa, rose hips, nettles, Dong Quai, watercress, dandelions, seaweeds, and wild seeds. Depleted by mineral oil and sulphates.

• *Vitamin K.* Found in leafy greens, corn and soybean oils, liver, cereals, dairy products, meats, fruits, egg yolk, blackstrap molasses. Herbal sources: nettles, alfalfa, kelp, and green tea. Depleted by x-rays, radiation, air pollution, enemas, frozen foods, antibiotics, rancid fats, and aspirin.

• *Thiamine (vitamin B_1).* Found in asparagus, cauliflower, cabbage, kale, spirulina, seaweeds, and citrus. Herbal sources: peppermint, burdock, sage, yellow dock, alfalfa, red clover, fenugreek, raspberry leaves, nettles, catnip, watercress, yarrow, briar rose buds, and rose hips.

• *Riboflavin (vitamin B_2).* Found in beans, greens, onions, seaweeds, spirulina, dairy products, and mushrooms. Herbal sources: peppermint, alfalfa, parsley, echinacea, yellow dock, hops, dandelion, ginseng, dulse, kelp, and fenugreek.

• *Pyridoxine (B_2).* Found in baked potato with skin, broccoli, prunes, bananas, dried beans and lentils; all meats, poultry, and fish.

• *Folic acid (B factor).* Found in liver, eggs, leafy greens, yeast, legumes, whole grains, nuts, fruits (bananas, orange juice, grapefruit juice), and vegetables (broccoli, spinach, asparagus, brussels sprouts). Herbal sources: nettles, alfalfa, parsley, sage, catnip, peppermint, plantain, comfrey leaves, and chickweed.

• *Niacin (B factor)*. Found in grains, meats, and nuts, and especially asparagus, spirulina, cabbage, and bee pollen. Herbal sources: hops, raspberry leaves, red clover, slippery elm, echinacea, licorice, rose hips, nettles, alfalfa, and parsley.

• *Bioflavonoids*. Found in citrus pulp and rind. Herbal sources: buckwheat greens, blue-green algae, elderberries, hawthorn fruits, rose hips, horsetail, and shepherd's purse.

• *Carotenes*. Found in carrots, cabbage, winter squash, sweet potatoes, dark leafy greens, apricots, spirulina, and seaweeds. Herbal sources: peppermint, yellow dock, uva ursi, parsley, alfalfa, raspberry leaves, nettles, dandelion greens, kelp, green onions, violet leaves, cayenne, paprika, lamb's quarters, sage, peppermint, chickweed, horsetail, black cohosh, and rose hips.

• *Essential fatty acids (EFAs), including GLA, omega-6, and omega-3*. Found in safflower oil and wheat germ oil. Herbal sources: all wild plants contain EFAs. Commercial sources: flaxseed oil, evening primrose, black currant, and borage.

• *Boron*. Found in organic fruits, vegetables, and nuts. Herbal sources: all organic weeds, including chickweed, purslane, nettles, dandelion, and yellow dock.

• *Calcium*. Found in milk and dairy products, leafy greens, broccoli, clams, oysters, almonds, walnuts, sunflower seeds, sesame seeds (tahini), legumes, tofu; softened bones of canned fish (sardines, mackerel, salmon); seaweed vegetables, whole grains, whey, and shellfish. Herbal sources: valerian, kelp, nettles, horsetail, peppermint, sage, uva ursi, yellow dock, chickweed, red clover, oatstraw, parsley, black currant leaves, raspberry leaves, plantain leaves/seeds, borage, dandelion leaves, amaranth leaves, and lamb's quarter. Depleted by coffee, sugar, salt, alcohol, cortisone enemas, and too much phosphorus.

• *Chromium*. Found in barley grass, bee pollen, prunes, nuts, mushrooms, liver, beets, and whole wheat. Herbal sources: oatstraw, nettles, red clover, catnip, dulse, wild yam, yarrow, horsetail, black cohosh, licorice, echinacea, valerian, and sarsaparilla. Depleted by white sugar.

- *Copper.* Found in liver, shellfish, nuts, legumes, water, organically grown grains, leafy greens, seaweeds, and bittersweet chocolate. Herbal sources: skullcap, sage, horsetail, and chickweed.

- *Iron.* (Heme iron is easily absorbed by the body; nonheme iron is not as easily absorbed, so it should be taken with vitamin C.) Heme iron is found in liver, meat, and poultry; nonheme iron is found in dried fruit, seeds, almonds, cashews, enriched and whole grains, legumes, and leafy green vegetables. Herbal sources: chickweed, kelp, burdock, catnip, horsetail, Althea root, milk thistle seed, uva ursi, dandelion leaves/root, yellow dock root, Dong Quai, black cohosh, echinacea, plantain leaves, sarsaparilla, nettles, peppermint, licorice, valerian, and fenugreek. Depleted by coffee, black tea, enemas, alcohol, aspirin, carbonated drinks, lack of protein, and too much dairy.

- *Magnesium.* Found in leafy greens, seaweeds, nuts, whole grains, yogurt, cheese, potatoes, corn, peas, and squash. Herbal sources: oatstraw, licorice, kelp, nettle, dulse, burdock, chickweed, Althea root, horsetail, sage, raspberry leaves, red clover, valerian, yellow dock, dandelion, carrot tops, parsley, and evening primrose. Depleted by alcohol, chemical diuretics, enemas, antibiotics, and excessive fat intake.

- *Manganese.* Found in any leaf or seed from a plant grown in healthy soil, and seaweeds. Herbal sources: raspberry leaves, uva ursi, chickweed, milk thistle, yellow dock, ginseng, wild yam, hops, catnip, echinacea, horsetail, kelp, nettles, and dandelion.

- *Molybdenum.* Found in organically raised dairy products, legumes, grains, and leafy greens. Herbal sources: nettles, dandelion greens, sage, oatstraw, fenugreek, raspberry leaves, red clover, horsetail, chickweed, and seaweeds.

- *Nickel.* Found in chocolate, nuts, dried beans, and cereals. Herbal sources: alfalfa, red clover, oatstraw, and fenugreek.

- *Phosphorus.* Found in whole grains, seeds, and nuts. Herbal sources: peppermint, yellow dock, milk thistle, fennel, hops, chickweed, nettles, dandelion, parsley, dulse, and red clover. Depleted by antacids.

- *Potassium*. Found in celery, cabbage, peas, parsley, broccoli, peppers, carrots, potato skins, eggplant, whole grains, pears, citrus, and seaweeds. Herbal sources: sage, catnip, hops, dulse, peppermint, skullcap, kelp, red clover, horsetail, nettles, borage, and plantain. Depleted by coffee, sugar, salt, alcohol, enemas, vomiting, diarrhea, chemical diuretics, and dieting.

- *Selenium*. Found in dairy products, seaweeds, grains, garlic, liver, kidneys, fish, and shellfish. Herbal sources: catnip, milk thistle, valerian, dulse, black cohosh, ginseng, uva ursi, hops, echinacea, kelp, raspberry leaves, rose buds and hips, hawthorn berries, fenugreek, sarsaparilla, and yellow dock.

- *Silicon*. Found in unrefined grains, root vegetables, spinach, and leeks. Herbal sources: horsetail, dulse, echinacea, cornsilk, burdock, oatstraw, licorice, chickweed, uva ursi, and sarsaparilla.

- *Sulfur*. Found in eggs, dairy products, cabbage family plants, onions, garlic, parsley, and watercress. Herbal sources: nettles, sage, plantain, and horsetail.

- *Zinc*. Found in oysters, seafood, meat, liver, eggs, whole grains, wheat germ, pumpkin seeds, and spirulina. Herbal sources: skullcap, sage, wild yam, chickweed, echinacea, nettles, dulse, milk thistle, and sarsaparilla. Depleted by alcohol and air pollution.

Carbohydrates and Fatigue

One of the most important factors in combating fatigue is maintaining normal blood sugar levels. Many people suffer from repeated episodes of low blood sugar, known as *hypoglycemia*. This is usually caused by consuming too many carbohydrates, which produces an initial "rush" of energy, followed by a tremendous "crash," sometimes known as postprandial depression (or postmeal depression). When you're hypothyroid, it's not at all unusual to crave simple carbohydrates, such as sugars and sweets. The simpler the carbohydrate, the faster it breaks down into glucose, and the faster the drop in blood sugar, leading to a drop in energy levels and mood.

If you think you suffer from low blood sugar, schedule an appointment with a nutritionist through your primary care physician and plan a diet that is based on a variety of foods, rather than one that is mostly carbohydrates. By increasing your intake of protein and fiber, you can help to delay the breakdown of your food into glucose, which will keep your blood sugar levels more stable throughout the day.

Supplements

Hypothyroidism can cause you to become depleted in vitamins and minerals. You may benefit from the following supplements:

- Beta-carotene 10,000–25,000 IUs
- Bioflavonoids 250–500 mg
- Biotin 150–500 mcg
- Calcium 600–1,000 mg
- Chromium 200–400 mcg
- Copper 2–3 mg
- Folic acid 500–1,000 mcg
- Hydrochloric acid (with meals, for chronic stress) 5–10 grains
- Inositol 500–1,000 mg
- Iodine 150–200 mcg
- Iron (menstruating women especially) 10–20 mg
- L-amino acids (L-glutamine, L-tyrosine, L-phenylalanine, and L-tryptophan) 1,000–1,500 mg
- L-cysteine 250–500 mg (take with vitamin C)
- Magnesium 350–600 mg (an Epsom salt bath is also magnesium)
- Manganese 5–10 mg
- Molybdenum 300–800 mg
- PABA 50–100 mg
- Pancreatic enzymes (after meals) 1–2 tablets
- Pantothenic acid (B_5) 500–1,000 mg
- Potassium 300–500 mg
- Pyridoxal-5-phosphate 25–75 mg
- Selenium 200–400 mcg
- Sulfur (check with your doctor or pharmacist about RDI)
- Superoxide dismutase (enzyme—check with your doctor or pharmacist about RDI)
- Thiamine (B_1) 75–150 mg

- Vitamin A 7,500–15,000 IUs
- Vitamin D 400 IUs
- Vitamin E 400–1,000 IUs
- Vitamin K 200–400 mcg
- Water 2–3 qts
- Zinc 30–60 mg

Battling the Bulge

By reducing your bloat and improving your digestion, you're well on your way to reducing your weight. Add to that all the information in this next section, and you'll know more about managing weight problems than most people.

The Bad News About Low-Fat Diets

If you think the key to weight loss is avoiding fat, think again. There is new thinking about what many perceive to be the dangers of low-fat dieting. Not only do they *not* work according to many critics, but they promote insulin resistance. A low-fat diet is a diet where most of your calories come from carbohydrates rather than protein or fat. Carbohydrates convert into glucose quickly in the body. So you eat, feel full, and then feel very hungry again. In order to feel satisfied and satiated, we must have some fat in our diets. But in addition to this, fat in our diets also triggers fat-burning compounds in our bodies. Years of conditioning us to eat no fat has made most people fatter, and has dramatically increased our risk of developing Type 2 diabetes. This is because of the amount of insulin we require to "clean up" the carbohydrates that convert so quickly into sugar (see my books *50 Ways to Manage Type 2 Diabetes* or *The Type 2 Diabetic Woman*). And higher insulin levels—get this—increase your appetite.

There is now a whole industry of diet books promoting low-, or no-carbohydrate diets, such as *Dr. Atkins' New Diet Revolution*, *Protein Power*, and *The Zone*. But the diets promoted in these books are considered by many nutrition experts to be dangerous. The Dr. Atkins diet is dangerous because it is based on a huge amount of saturated fat, the major source of "bad cholesterol" in the diet. Regardless of how much weight you may lose on the Atkins diet, you are still at risk for heart disease because of the saturated fat and high LDL (low-density lipids) levels. The Zone diet, according to some experts, has no scientific basis; the book claims that high carbs and insulin make you fat, when in fact it is calories from all sources of food that make you fat when you don't output the energy needed to burn them off. The best advice now is to limit carbohydrates in each meal to about 40 percent, and be sure to have about 30 percent protein and 30 percent of "helpful" fat (see further on). Some carbohydrates convert into glucose faster than others. Table 4.1 can help you select slower-converting carbohydrates to balance your diet.

Understanding Carbohydrates

It's important to understand what is meant by "carbohydrates." The diet lingo can often confuse us. Carbohydrates—starchy stuff, such as rice, pasta, breads, or potatoes—can be stored as fat when eaten in excess.

Carbohydrates can be simple or complex. Simple carbohydrates are found in any food that has natural sugar (honey, fruits, juices, vegetables, milk) and anything that contains table sugar.

Complex carbohydrates are more sophisticated foods that are made up of larger molecules, such as grain foods, starches, and foods high in fiber.

Normally, all carbs convert into glucose when you eat them (see Table 4.2). Glucose is the technical term for "simplest sugar." All your energy comes from glucose in your blood—also known as blood glucose or blood sugar—your body fuel. When your blood sugar is used up, you feel weak and tired . . . and hungry. But what happens when you eat more carbohydrates than your body can use? Your body will store those extra carbs as fat. What we also know is that the rate at which glucose is absorbed by your body from carbohydrates is affected by other parts of your meal, such as the protein, fiber, and fat. If you're eating only carbohydrates and no protein or fat, for example, they will

Table 4.1 The Glycemic Index at-a-Glance

This glycemic index, developed at the University of Toronto, measures the rate at which various foods convert to glucose, which is assigned a value of 100. Higher numbers indicate a more rapid conversion to glucose. This is not an exhaustive list and should be used as a *sample* only. This is not an index of food energy values or calories; some low GI foods are high in fat, while some high GI foods low in fat. Keep in mind, too, that these values differ depending upon what else you're eating with that food and how the food is prepared.

Sugars

Glucose = 100
Honey = 87
Table sugar = 59
Fructose = 20

Snacks

Mars bar = 68
Potato chips = 51
Sponge cake = 46
Fish sticks = 38
Tomato soup = 38
Sausages = 28
Peanuts = 13

Cereals

Cornflakes = 80
Shredded wheat = 67
Muesli = 66
All-Bran = 51
Oatmeal = 49

Breads

Whole wheat = 72
White = 69
Buckwheat = 51

Fruits

Raisins = 64
Banana = 62
Orange juice = 46
Orange = 40
Apple = 39

Dairy Products

Ice cream = 36
Yogurt = 36
Milk = 34
Skim milk = 32

Root Vegetables

Parsnips = 97
Carrots = 92
Instant mashed potatoes = 80
New boiled potato = 70
Beets = 64
Yam = 51
Sweet potato = 48

Pasta and Rice

White rice = 72
Brown rice = 66
Spaghetti (white) = 50
Spaghetti (whole wheat) = 42

Legumes

Frozen peas = 51
Baked beans = 40
Chickpeas = 36
Lima beans = 36
Butter beans = 36
Black-eyed peas = 33
Green beans = 31
Kidney beans = 29
Lentils = 29
Dried soybeans = 15

Table 4.2 How Your Food Breaks Down

Many foods are a combination of carbs, protein, and fats. Here is a breakdown of how the various components of your meal break down.

Complex Carbohydrates (digests more slowly)

fruits*
vegetables* (corn, potatoes, etc.)
grains (breads, pastas, and cereals)
legumes (dried beans, peas, and lentils)

*Note: Many vegetables and herbs have no significant effect on your blood sugar levels. These include artichokes, asparagus, mushrooms, bean sprouts, okra, onions, parsley, peppers, radish, celery, rapini, cucumber, shallots, eggplant, endive, tomato, kohlrabi, and zucchini.

Simple Carbohydrates (digests quickly)

fruits/fruit juices*
sugars (sucrose, fructose, etc.)
honey
corn syrup
sorghum
date sugar
molasses
lactose

*Note: Lemon and lime juice do not have a significant effect on blood sugar levels, nor do artificial sweeteners, and clear coffee or tea.

Proteins (digests slowly)

lean meats
fatty meats
poultry
fish
eggs
low-fat cheese
high-fat cheese
legumes
grains

Fats (digest slowly)

high-fat dairy products (butter or cream)
oils (canola/corn/olive/safflower/sunflower)
lard
avocados
olives
nuts
fatty meats

(continued on next page)

Table 4.1 The Glycemic Index at-a-Glance (continued)

Fiber (doesn't digest; goes through you)

whole-grain breads
cereals (e.g., oatmeal)
all fruits
legumes (beans and lentils)
leafy greens
cruciferous vegetables

Source: "How Your Food Breaks Down" copyright 1997, 1999, 2001, M. Sara Rosenthal.

convert into glucose more quickly—to the point where you may feel mood swings, as your blood sugar rises and dips.

Understanding Sugar

Sugars are found naturally in many foods you eat. The simplest form of sugar is glucose, which is what blood sugar, also called blood glucose, is—your basic body fuel. You can buy pure glucose at any drugstore in the form of dextrose tablets. Dextrose is just "edible glucose." For example, when you see people having "sugar water" fed to them intravenously, dextrose is the sugar in that water. When you see "dextrose" on a candy bar label, it means that the candy bar manufacturer used "edible glucose" in the recipe.

Glucose is the baseline ingredient of all naturally occurring sugars, which include:

- *Sucrose:* table or white sugar, naturally found in sugar cane and sugar beets
- *Fructose:* the natural sugar in fruits and vegetables
- *Lactose:* the natural sugar in all milk products
- *Maltose:* the natural sugar in grains (flours and cereals)

When you ingest a natural sugar of any kind, you're actually ingesting one part glucose, and one or two parts of *another* naturally occurring sugar. For example, sucrose is biochemically constructed from one part glucose and one part fructose. So . . . from glucose it came, and unto glucose it shall return—once it hits your digestive system. The same is true for all naturally occurring sugars, with the exception of lactose. As it happens, lactose breaks down into glucose and an "odd duck" simple sugar, galactose (which I used to think was something in our solar system until I became a health writer). Just think of lactose as the "milky way" and you'll probably remember.

Simple sugars can get pretty complicated when you discuss their molecular structures. For example, simple sugars can be classified as monosaccharides (aka "single sugars") or dissaccharides (aka double sugars). But unless you're writing a chemistry exam on sugars, you don't need to know this confusing stuff: you just need to know that all naturally occurring sugars wind up as glucose once you eat them; glucose is carried to your cells through the bloodstream and is used as body fuel or energy.

How long does it take for one of the above sugars to return to glucose? Well, it greatly depends on the amount of fiber in your food, how much protein you've eaten, and how much fat accompanies the sugar in your meal. If you have enough energy or fuel, once that sugar becomes glucose, it can be stored as fat. And that's how—and why—sugar can make you fat.

Factory-Added Sugars

What you have to watch out for is *added sugar*; these are sugars that manufacturers add to foods during processing or packaging. Foods containing fruit juice concentrates, invert sugar, regular corn syrup, honey, molasses, hydrolyzed lactose syrup, or high-fructose corn syrup (made from highly concentrated fructose through the hydrolysis of starch) all have added sugars. Many people don't realize, however, that pure, *unsweetened* fruit juice is still a potent source of sugar, even when it contains no added sugar. Extra lactose (naturally occurring sugar in milk products), dextrose ("edible glucose"), and maltose (naturally occurring sugar in grains) are also contained in many of your foods. In other words, the products may have naturally occurring sugars anyway, and then *more* sugar is thrown in to enhance consistency, taste, and so on. The best way to know how much sugar is in a product is to look at the nutritional label for "carbohydrates."

Understanding Fat

Fat is technically known as *fatty acids*, which are crucial nutrients for our cells. We cannot live without fatty acids, or fat. If you looked at each fat molecule carefully, you'd find three different kinds of fatty acids on it: saturated (solid), monounsaturated (less solid, with the exception of olive and peanut oils), and polyunsaturated (liquid) fatty acids. When you see the term "unsaturated fat," this refers to either monounsaturated or polyunsaturated fats.

These three fatty acids combine with glycerol to make what's chemically known as triglycerides. Each fat molecule is a link chain made up of glycerol, carbon atoms, and hydrogen atoms. The more hydrogen atoms on that chain, the more saturated or solid the fat. The liver breaks down fat molecules by secreting bile (stored in the gallbladder—its sole function). The liver also makes cholesterol. Too much saturated fat may cause your liver to overproduce cholesterol, while the triglycerides in your bloodstream will rise, perpetuating the problem.

Fat is therefore a good thing—in moderation. Fat in the diet comes from meats, dairy products, and vegetable oils. Other sources of fat include coconuts (60 percent fat), peanuts (78 percent fat), and avocados (82 percent fat). There are different kinds of fatty acids in these sources of fats: saturated, monounsaturated, and polyunsaturated (which, again, is what is meant by the term "unsaturated fat"). And then there is a fourth kind of fat in our diets: transfatty acids. This is a factory-made fat that is found in margarines, for example.

To cut through all this big, fat jargon, you can boil down fat into two categories: "harmful fats" and "helpful fats" (which the popular press often defines as "good fats/bad fats").

Harmful Fats

The following are harmful fats because they can increase your risk of cardiovascular problems, as well as many cancers, including colon and breast cancers. These are fats that are fine in moderation, but harmful in excess (and harmless if not eaten at all):

• *Saturated fats*. These are solid at room temperature and stimulate cholesterol production in your body. In fact, the way that saturated fat looks prior to your ingesting it is the way it will look when it lines your arteries. Foods high in saturated fat include processed meat, fatty meat, lard, butter, margarine, solid vegetable shortening, chocolate, and tropical oils (coconut oil is more than 90 percent saturated). Saturated fat should be consumed only in very low amounts.

• *Transfatty acids.* These are factory-made fats that behave just like saturated fat in your body. See further on for details.

Helpful Fats

These fats are beneficial to your health and actually protect against certain health problems, such as cardiovascular disease. These are fats that you are encouraged to use more, rather than less, frequently in your diet. In fact, nutritionists suggest that you substitute harmful fats with these.

• *Unsaturated fat.* This is partially solid or liquid at room temperature. The more liquid the fat, the more polyunsaturated it is, which, in fact, *lowers* your cholesterol levels. This group of fats includes monounsaturated fats and polyunsaturated fats. Sources of unsaturated fats include vegetable oils (canola, safflower, sunflower, corn) and seeds and nuts. Unsaturated fats come from plants, with the exception of tropical oils, such as coconut.

• *Fish fats (aka omega-3 oils).* The fats naturally present in fish that swim in cold waters, known as omega-3 fatty acids or fish oils, are all polyunsaturated. Again, polyunsaturated fats are good for you: they lower cholesterol levels, are crucial for brain tissue, and protect against heart disease. Look for cold water fish such as mackerel, albacore tuna, salmon, and sardines.

Factory-Made Fats

An assortment of factory-made fats have been introduced into our diet, courtesy of food producers who are trying to give us the taste of fat without all the calories of saturated fats. Unfortunately, man-made fats offer their own bag of horrors. That's because when a fat is made in a factory, it becomes a "transfatty acid," a harmful fat that *not only* raises the level of "bad" cholesterol (LDL, short for low-density lipids) in your bloodstream, but lowers the amount of "good" cholesterol (HDL, short for high-density lipids) that's already there.

How, exactly, does a "transfatty acid" come into being? Transfatty acids are what you get when you make a liquid oil, such as corn oil, into a more solid or spreadable substance, such as margarine. Transfatty acids, you might say, are the "road to hell, paved with good intentions." Someone, way back when, thought that if you could take the "good fat"—unsaturated fat—and solidify it, so it could double as butter or lard, you could eat the same things without missing the spreadable fat. That sounds like a great idea. Unfortunately, to make an unsaturated liquid fat more solid, you have to add hydrogen to its molecules. This is known as *hydrogenation*, the process that converts liquid fat to semisolid fat. That ever-popular candy bar ingredient, "hydrogenated palm oil" is a classic example of a transfatty acid. Hydrogenation also prolongs the shelf life of a fat, such as polyunsaturated fats, which can oxidize when exposed to air, causing rancid odors or flavors. Deep-frying oils used in the restaurant trade are generally hydrogenated.

Transfatty acid is sold as a polyunsaturated or monounsaturated fat with a line of advertising copy such as: "Made from polyunsaturated vegetable oil." Except in your body, it is treated as a *saturated* fat. So really, transfatty acids are a saturated fat in disguise. The advertiser may, in fact, say that the product contains "no saturated fat" or is "healthier" than the comparable animal or tropical oil product with saturated fat. So be careful out there: *read your labels*. The magic word you're looking for is "hydrogenated." If the product lists a variety of unsaturated fats (monounsaturated X oil, polyunsaturated Y oil, and so on), keep reading. If the word hydrogenated appears, count that product as a saturated fat; your body will!

Margarine Versus Butter

There's an old tongue twister: "Betty Botter bought some butter that made the batter bitter; so Betty Botter bought more butter that made the batter better." Are we making our batters bitter or better with margarine? It depends.

Since the news of transfatty acids broke in the late 1980s, margarine manufacturers began to offer some less "bitter" margarines; some contain no hydrogenated oils, while others contain much smaller amounts. Margarines with less than 60 to 80 percent oil (9 to 11 grams of fat) will contain 1.0 to 3.0 grams of transfatty acids per serving, compared to butter, which is 53 percent saturated fat. You might say it's a choice between a bad fat and a *worse* fat.

It's also possible for a liquid vegetable oil to retain a high concentration of unsaturated fat when it's been partially hydrogenated. In this case, your body will metabolize this as some saturated fat and some unsaturated fat.

Fake Fat

We have artificial sweeteners; why not artificial fat? This question has led to the creation of an emerging yet highly suspicious ingredient: *fat substitutes*, designed to replace real fat and hence reduce the calories from real fat without compromising the taste. This is done by creating a fake fat that the body cannot absorb.

One of the first fat substitutes was Simplesse, an All-Natural Fat Substitute, made from milk and egg-white protein, which was developed by the NutraSweet Company. Simplesse apparently adds 1 to 2 calories per gram instead of the usual 9 calories per gram from fat. Other fat substitutes simply take protein and carbohydrates and modify them in some way to simulate the textures of fat (creamy, smooth, and so on). All of these fat substitutes help to create low-fat products.

The calorie-free fat substitute currently being promoted is called olestra, developed by Procter and Gamble. It's available in the United States in a variety of savory snacks such as potato chips and crackers. Olestra is a potentially dangerous ingredient that most experts feel can do more harm than good. Canada has not yet approved it.

Olestra is made from a combination of vegetable oils and sugar. Therefore, it tastes just like the real thing, but the biochemical structure is a molecule too big for your liver to break down. So, olestra just gets passed into the large intestine and is excreted. Olestra is more than an "empty" molecule, however. According to the FDA Commissioner of Food and Drugs, olestra may cause diarrhea and cramps and may deplete your body of vital nutrients, including vitamins A, D, E, and

K, necessary for blood to clot. And indeed, all studies conducted by Procter and Gamble have shown this potential. If the FDA approves olestra for use as a cooking-oil substitute, you'll see it in every imaginable high-fat product. But there is another danger with olestra, which nutritionists raised in a critique of olestra in a 1996 issue of *The University of California at Berkeley Wellness Letter* (the year olestra was approved for test markets). Instead of encouraging people to choose nutritious foods, such as fruits, grains, and vegetables over high-fat foods, products like these encourage a high *fake*-fat diet that's still too low in fiber and other essential nutrients. And the no-fat icing on the cake is that these people could potentially wind up with a vitamin deficiency, to boot. Products like olestra should make you nervous.

Reading Food Labels

Since 1993, food labels have been adhering to strict guidelines set out by the Food and Drug Administration (FDA) and the U.S. Department of Agriculture's (USDA) Food Safety and Inspection Service (FSIS). All labels will list "Nutrition Facts" on the side or back of the package. The "Percent Daily Values" column tells you how high or low that food is in various nutrients, such as fat, saturated fat, and cholesterol. A number of 5 or less is "low"—good news if the product shows <5 for fat, saturated fat, and cholesterol, bad news if the product is <5 for fiber. Serving sizes are also confusing. Foods that are similar are given the same *type* of serving size defined by the FDA. That means that five cereals that all weigh X grams per cup will share the same serving size.

Calories (how much energy) and calories from fat (how much fat) are also listed per serving of food. Total carbohydrate, dietary fiber, sugars, other carbohydrates (which means starches), total fat, saturated fat, cholesterol, sodium, potassium, and vitamins and minerals are given in Percent Daily Values, based on the 2,000-calorie diet recommended by the U.S. government.

But that's not where the confusion ends—*or even begins*! You have to wade through the various "claims" and understand what they mean. For example, anything that is "X-free" (as in sugar-free, saturated fat–free, cholesterol-free, sodium-free, calorie-free, and so on) means that the product indeed has "no X" or that "X" is so tiny, it is dietarily insignificant. This is not the same thing as a label that says "95 percent fat-free." In this case, the product contains relatively small amounts of fat, but it still has fat. This claim is based on 100 grams of the product. For example, if a snack food contains 2.5 grams of fat per 50 grams, it can be said to be "95 percent fat-free."

A label that screams "low in saturated fat" or "low in calories" is *not* fat-free or calorie-free. It means that you can eat a large amount of that food without exceeding the Daily Value for that food. In potato-chip country, that could mean you can eat twelve potato chips instead of six. So if you eat the whole bag of "low-fat" chips, you're still eating a lot of fat. Be sure to check serving sizes.

"Cholesterol-free" or "low-cholesterol" means that the product doesn't have any, or much, animal fat (hence, cholesterol). This doesn't mean "low-fat." Pure vegetable oil doesn't come from animals but is pure fat!

"Less and More"

And then there are the "comparison claims" such as "fewer," "reduced," "less," "more," or my favorite—"light" (or worse, "lite"!). These words appear on foods that have been nutritionally altered from a previous "version" or competitor's version. For example, *Brand X Potato Chips—Regular* may have much more fat than *Brand X Potato Chips Lite—"With Less Fat Than Regular Brand X."* That doesn't mean that *Brand X Lite* is fat-free, or even low in fat. It just means it's some percent *lower* in fat than *Brand X Regular.*

On the flip side, *Brand Y* may have a trace amount of calcium, while *Brand Y—"Now With More Calcium"* may still have a small amount of calcium, but 10 percent more than *Brand Y.* (In other words, you may still need to eat 100 bowls of *Brand Y* before you get the daily requirement for calcium!)

To be light (or "lite"), a product has to contain either one-third fewer calories or half the fat of the regular product. Or, a low-calorie or low-fat food contains 50 percent less sodium. Something that is "light in sodium" means it has at least 50 percent less sodium than the regular product, such as canned soup. (But if you're buying hair color that reads "light brown," it is a descriptive word, not referring to an ingredient!)

"Sugar-Free"

When a label says "sugar-free," it contains less than 0.5 grams of sugar per serving, while a "reduced-sugar" food contains at least 25 percent less sugar per serving than the regular product. If the label also states that the product is not a reduced- or low-calorie food, or it is not for weight control, it's got enough sugar in there to make you think twice.

But sugar-free in the language of labels simply means "sucrose-free." That doesn't mean the product is *carbohydrate free*, as in dextrose-free, lactose-free, glucose-free, or fructose-free. Check the labels for all things ending in "-ose" to find out the sugar content; you're not just looking for sucrose. Watch out for "no added sugar," "without added sugar," or "no sugar added." This simply means: "We didn't put the sugar in, God did."

Reading Dairy Labels

If you're battling the bulge, it's important to know how much saturated fat is in your dairy purchases.

- Whole milk is made up of 48 percent calories from fat.
- 2 percent milk gets 37 percent of its calories from fat.
- 1 percent milk gets 26 percent of its calories from fat.
- Skim milk is completely fat-free.
- Cheese gets 50 percent of its calories from fat, unless it's skim milk cheese.
- Butter gets 95 percent of its calories from fat.
- Yogurt gets 15 percent of its calories from fat.

5

The Hypothyroid Active Living Program

WHEN MANAGING HYPOTHYROIDISM, you need to move. The fatigue, lethargy, and depression that accompanies bouts of hypothyroidism makes moving our bodies the last thing we want to do. This chapter will help you find ways to move without "exercising." The word *exercise* for many is intimidating, and conjures up images of having to go to a fitness class or club. The Oxford dictionary defines exercise as "the exertion of muscles, limbs, etc., especially for health's sake; bodily, mental, or spiritual training." In the Western world, we have placed an emphasis on "bodily training" when we talk about exercise, completely ignoring mental and spiritual health, which includes meditation and deep breathing. People also think of exercise as being limited to Western sports or solo activities, such as jogging. This chapter will show you a range of alternative activities to the usual "fitness club/jogging" model that few people enjoy. All you have to do is choose one activity in this chapter to complement the diet advice in the previous chapter, and you will feel better regardless of whether you're balanced on thyroid medication or not.

Creating More Oxygen

If you look up the word *aerobic* in the dictionary, what you'll find is the chemistry definition: "living in free oxygen." Aerobic exercises are designed to create faster breathing, so we can take more oxygen into our bodies. *Why are we doing this?* Because the blood contains *oxygen*! The faster your blood flows, the more oxygen can flow to your organs. When your heart beats faster, it gets a "workout" of sorts, which is usually good for the heart, unless you have a condition that affects your heart.

When more oxygen is in our bodies, we burn fat (see further on), our breathing improves, our blood pressure improves, and our hearts work better—which benefits our entire body, leading to regularity, for example. Oxygen also lowers triglycerides and cholesterol, increasing our high-density lipoproteins (HDL) or the "good" cholesterol, while decreasing our low-density lipoproteins (LDL) or the "bad" cholesterol. This means that your arteries will unclog and you may significantly decrease your risk of heart disease and stroke. More oxygen makes our brains work better, which helps to combat the brain fog of hypothyroidism. Studies show that depression is decreased when we increase oxygen flow into our bodies, too, another effect of hypothyroidism. Ancient techniques such as yoga, which specifically improve mental and spiritual well-being, achieve this by combining deep breathing and stretching, which improves oxygen and blood flow to specific parts of the body.

Oxygen also burns fat. If you were to go to your fridge and pull out some animal fat (chicken skin, red-meat fat, or butter), throw it in the sink, and light it with a match, it will burn. What makes the flame yellow is oxygen; what fuels the fire is the fat. That same process goes on in your body. The oxygen will burn your fat; however, you increase the oxygen flow in your body through jumping around/increasing your heart rate or employing an established deep-breathing technique.

You can increase the flow of oxygen into your bloodstream without exercising your heart muscle, by learning how to breathe deeply through your diaphragm. There are many yogalike programs and videos available that can teach you this technique, which does not require you to jump around. The benefit is that you would be increasing the oxygen flow into your bloodstream, which is better than doing nothing at all to improve your health, and has many health benefits, according to a myriad of wellness practitioners. Deep breathing exercises can also help to strengthen digestion and keep you regular.

The phrase "aerobic activity" means that the *activity* causes your heart to pump harder and faster, and causes you to breathe faster, which increases oxygen flow. Activities such as cross-country skiing, walking, hiking, and biking are all aerobic. But you know what? Exercise practitioners hate the terms "aerobic activity" or "aerobics program" because it is not about what people do in their daily lives. Health promoters are replacing these terms with the phrase "active living"—because that's what becoming unsedentary is all about. Here are some starter tips.

- If you drive everywhere, pick the parking space farther away from your destination so you can work some daily walking into your life.

- If you take public transit everywhere, get off one or two stops early so you can walk the rest of the way to your destination.

- Choose stairs over escalators or elevators.

- Park at one side of the mall, then walk to the other.

- Take a stroll after dinner around your neighborhood.

- Volunteer to walk a dog (could be a neighbor's, a friend's, or your own!).

- On weekends, go to the zoo or get out to flea markets, garage sales, and so on.

Becoming More Active

If you do roughly twenty minutes of exercise less than once a week, you're relatively sedentary. If you've been sedentary most of your life, there's nothing wrong with starting off with simple, even leisurely, activities such as gardening, feeding the birds in a park, or a few simple stretches. Any step you make toward being more active is a crucial and important step. Experts also recommend that you find a friend, neighbor, or relative to get physical with you. When your activity plans include someone else, you'll be less apt to cancel plans or to make excuses for not getting out there.

Choose an activity that's right for you. Whether it's walking, chopping wood, jumping rope, or folk dancing—pick something you *enjoy*. You don't have to do the same thing each time, either. Vary your routine to avoid monotony. Just make sure that whatever activity you choose is continuous for the duration. Walking for two minutes, then stopping for three isn't continuous. It's also important to choose an activity that doesn't aggravate a preexisting health problem. Try not to let two days pass without doing something. And pick a duration. If you're very fatigued as a result of your hypothyroidism, even a few minutes helps. See Table 5.1 for some suggestions.

Weight-Bearing Activities

The following are weight-bearing activities, which help build bone mass:

- Walking
- Running
- Jogging
- Bicycling
- Hiking
- Tai chi
- Cross-country skiing
- Gardening
- Weightlifting
- Snowshoeing
- Climbing stairs
- Tennis
- Bowling
- Rowing
- Dancing
- Water workouts
- Badminton
- Basketball
- Volleyball
- Soccer

Jogging

If you're someone who prefers jogging, here are some variations.

- After warming up with a fifteen-minute walk, simply walk quickly with maximum exertion for two minutes, then slow down for one minute. Keep your heart rate up on the downhill portion of a walk or a hike by adding lunges or squats.

Table 5.1 Traditional Activities

More Intense	Less Intense
Skiing	Golf
Running	Bowling
Jogging	Badminton
Stair-stepping or stair-climbing	Croquet
Trampolining	Sailing
Jumping rope	Swimming
Fitness walking	Strolling
Race walking	Stretching
Aerobics classes	
Roller skating	
Ice skating	
Biking	
Tennis	
Swimming	
Dancing (*any* kind will do, including tribal dances and folk dances)	

• Vary the way you walk for coordination and balance. Try lifting the knees as high as you can, as if marching. Alternate with a shuffle, letting the tips of your fingers touch the ground as you walk. Do a sideways "crab" walk. To strengthen the rarely used muscles of the ankles and feet, walk first on the outsides, then on the insides of your feet. Or practice walking backward.

Water Workouts

These are activities you can do in your local community pool.

• Start by walking in water that's relatively shallow (waist- or chest-deep). Your breathing and heartbeat will determine how hard you are working. Since you'll be moving fairly slowly, pay attention to your body.

• For all-over leg toning, take fifty steps forward, fifty steps sideways in crablike fashion, fifty steps backward, then fifty steps to the other side.

• To tone your arms, submerge yourself from the neck down, bringing the arms in and out as if clapping. The water will provide natural resistance.

• Deep-water workouts are the most difficult, because every move you make is met with resistance. Wear a flotation vest and run without touching the bottom for optimum exertion and little or no impact.

• You may also want to try buoyant ankle cuffs and styrofoam dumbbells or kickboards for full-body conditioning in the water.

Stretch

Ever watch a cat in action? Cats will never do anything before stretching. If stretching *is* your exercise, that's just fine; but if it's not the focus of your activity, do some stretching before and after you get really active to reduce muscle tightness. Here are three easy stretches anyone can incorporate into his or her day.

• *Shoulder rotations.* While breathing deeply and slowly, use a circular pattern to move the right shoulder, then switch to the left. One minute per shoulder is a good start.

• *Upper-back stretch.* Done sitting or standing, simply stretch your arms upward and slightly behind you, taking deep, slow breaths. With arms up, face your palms toward heaven and rotate your thumbs.

• *Arm circles.* Done sitting or standing, extend your arms so you look like a cross, then move your arms in circles, starting small and getting larger. (You know this one!)

Borg's Rate of Perceived Exertion (RPE)

This is a way of measuring activity intensity without finding your pulse, and because of its simplicity, it is now the recommended method for judging exertion. This Borg "scale" as it's dubbed goes from 6 to 20. An extremely light activity may rate a "7" for example, while a very,

very hard activity may rate a "19." What exercise practitioners recommend is that you do a "talk test" to rate your exertion. If you can't
talk without gasping for air, you may be working too hard. You should
be able to carry on a normal conversation throughout your activity.
What's crucial to remember about RPE is that it is extremely individual; what one person judges a "7," another may judge a "10."

Nontraditional Activities

The activities above are what I would define as traditionally "Western"
activities. But you may prefer some non-Western activities.

Yoga

Yoga is not just about stretches or postures, but is a way of life for
many. It is part of a whole science of living known as the Ayurveda.
The Ayurveda is an ancient Indian approach to health and wellness that
has stood up quite well to the test of time. It's roughly three thousand
years old. Essentially, it divides the universe into three basic constitu-
tions or "energies" known as doshas. The three doshas are based on
wind (Vata), fire (Pitta), and earth (Kapha). These doshas also govern
our bodies, personalities, and activities. When our doshas are balanced,
all functions well, but when they are not balanced, a state of disease
(disease as in "not at ease") can set in. Finding the balance involves
changing your diet to suit your predominant dosha (foods are classified as kapha, vata, or pitta and we eat more or less of whatever we
need for balance). Practicing yoga is a preventive health science that
involves certain physical postures, exercises, and meditations. Essentially, yoga is the "exercise" component of Ayurveda. It involves relaxing meditation, breathing, and physical postures designed to tone and
soothe your mental and physical state. Most people benefit from intro-
ductory yoga classes or videos.

Qi Gong

Every morning, all over China, people of all ages gather at parks to do
their daily qi gong exercises. Pronounced "chi kung," these are exercises that help get your life force energy (called the qi or "chi" in Chi-

nese) flowing and unblocked. Qi gong exercises are modeled after movements in wildlife (birds or animals), movement of trees, and other things in nature. The exercises have a continuous flow, rather than the stillness of a posture seen in yoga. Using the hands in various positions to gather in the qi, move the qi, or release the qi are the most important aspects of qi gong movements.

One of the first group of qi gong exercises you might learn are the "seasons"—Fall, Winter, Spring, Summer, and Late Summer (there are five seasons here). These exercises look like a dance with precise, slow movements. The word *qi* means vitality, energy, and life force; the word *gong* means practice, cultivate, refine. The Chinese believe that practicing qi gong balances the body, and improves physical and mental well-being. These exercises push the life force energy into the various meridian pathways that correspond to organs. It is the same map used in pressure point healing. Qi gong improves oxygen flow and enhances the lymphatic system. Qi gong is similar to tai chi, except it allows for greater flexibility in routine. The best way to learn qi gong is through a qualified instructor. You can generally find qi gong classes through the alternative healing community. Check health food stores and other centers that offer classes such as yoga or tai chi. Qi gong is difficult to learn from a book or video. An instructor is best.

6

The Hypothyroid Herbal and Wellness Program

THE INFORMATION IN this chapter is designed to complement your diet, activity program, and thyroid medication. There are a number of herbal remedies for many of the hypothyroid ailments such as fatigue, brain fog, and bloating. Hands-on healing strategies can also help with many hypothyroid symptoms. Coping with hypothyroidism, or any illness, is very stressful. By lowering your stress, you can also improve your overall health and sense of well being. A little self-care when you're hypothyroid goes a long way, too.

Herbs for Hypothyroidism

Many of the symptoms of hypothyroidism (see Chapter 1) can be alleviated with the aid of herbs. One of the symptoms most helped with herbal supplements is depression, which can be helped with the following:

St. John's Wort

Also known as *hypericum*, this has been used as a sort of "nerve tonic" in folk medicine for centuries. It's been shown to successfully treat mild to moderate depression, and anxiety. It's been used in Germany for years as a first-line treatment for depression, and is endorsed by the American Psychiatric Association. In Germany and other parts of

Europe, it outsells Prozac prescriptions. Since it was introduced into North America in the early 1990s, millions of North Americans have been successfully treated for depression with St. John's wort; in the United States, sales of St. John's wort and other botanical products reached an estimated $4.3 billion in 1998, according to *Nutrition Business Journal*. The benefits of St. John's wort are that it has minimal side effects, can be mixed with alcohol, is nonaddictive, and you don't need to increase your dose as you do with antidepressants. You can go on and off St. John's wort as you wish, without any problem; it helps you sleep and dream; it doesn't have any sedative effect, and, in fact, enhances your alertness.

Kava Root

From the black pepper family, another popular herb is kava (*Piper methysticum*). It has been a popular herbal drink in the South Pacific for centuries. Kava grows on the islands of Polynesia, and is known to calm nerves and ease stress, fatigue, and anxiety, which results in an antidepressant effect. Kava can also help alleviate migraine headaches and menstrual cramps. Placebo-controlled studies conducted by the National Institute of Mental Health showed that kava significantly relieved anxiety and stress, without the problem of dependency or addiction to the herb. Kava should not be combined with alcohol because it can make the effects of alcohol more potent. You should also check with your doctor before you combine kava with any prescription medications.

SAM-e

Pronounced "Sammy," this is another natural compound shown to help alleviate anxiety and mild depression. Since it was introduced in the United States in March 1999, more people have purchased Sam-e than St. John's wort. Sam-e has also been shown to help relieve joint pain and improve liver function, which makes it popular for people suffering from arthritis. Sam-e stands for S-adenosylmethionine, a compound made by your body's cells. Studies done in Italy during the 1970s documented Sam-e's effectiveness as an antidepressant; recent U.S. studies confirm the same results. Some people have reported hot, itchy ears as a side effect.

Inositol

This is a naturally occurring antidepressant that is present in many foods, such as vegetables, whole grains, milk, and meat, and should be available over the counter.

Phenylethylamine (PEA)

This is a nitrogen-containing compound found in small quantities in the brain. Studies show it works as a natural antidepressant.

Rubidium

Rubidium is a natural chemical in our bodies, belonging to the same family as lithium, potassium, and sodium. Studies show that it can work as an antidepressant.

Ginkgo

This is a plant used to treat a variety of ailments, and is a common herb in Chinese medicine. It can improve memory, and some studies show that it can boost the effectiveness of antidepressant medications.

Flower Power

One of the most popular natural emotional "rescues" people are turning to in droves are what's known as the Bach Flower remedies. The Bach flower remedies are thirty-eight homeopathically prepared plant and flower liquid extracts. Each flower remedy is designed to treat a different emotion. Dr. Edward Bach invented this healing tradition in the 1930s (during a time of extreme economic and social misery). Bach classified emotions into seven major groups (for example, fear, uncertainty, or loneliness) and thirty-eight different emotional states, and developed corresponding flower remedies. (See the list below.) These remedies work through homeopathic principles, stimulating the body's own capacity to heal itself. The flower remedies are made available as a liquid that is preserved in brandy. Taking the remedy involves diluting two drops of the pure liquid into 30 milliters of mineral water. You then take four drops of the dilution orally four times a day. You can also put two drops of the pure remedy into a glass of water, and just sip it throughout the day.

Rescue Remedy

Rescue remedy is a combination of five Bach flower remedies: Cherry Plum, Clematis, Impatiens, Rock Rose, and Star of Bethlehem. This combination works well for people who suffer from panic attacks or anxiety, and is designed to be taken pure, or "neat," from the bottle. You don't need to buy all of the Bach flower remedies and combine them yourself; Rescue remedy comes premixed. People can either take four drops of rescue remedy at once, orally, or dilute four drops in a glass of water and drink. Rescue Remedy reportedly works very quickly to calm the emotions.

The 38 Bach Flower Remedies

The following is a complete list of the bach flower remedies, and the corresponding emotional states they help to calm or quell.

- Agrimony: mental torture behind a cheerful face
- Aspen: fear of unknown things
- Beech: intolerance
- Centaury: the inability to say "no"
- Cerato: lack of trust in one's own decisions
- Cherry Plum: fear of the mind giving way
- Chestnut Bud: failure to learn from mistakes
- Chicory: selfish, possessive love
- Clematis: dreaming of the future without working in the present
- Crab Apple: the cleansing remedy, also for self-hatred
- Elm: overwhelmed by responsibility
- Gentian: discouragement after a setback
- Gorse: hopelessness and despair
- Heather: self-centeredness and self-concern
- Holly: hatred, envy, and jealousy
- Honeysuckle: living in the past
- Hornbeam: procrastination, tiredness at the thought of doing something
- Impatiens: impatience
- Larch: lack of confidence
- Mimulus: fear of known things

- Mustard: deep gloom for no reason
- Oak: the plodder who keeps going past the point of exhaustion
- Olive: exhaustion following mental or physical effort
- Pine: guilt
- Red Chestnut: over-concern for the welfare of loved ones
- Rock Rose: terror and fright
- Rock Water: self-denial, rigidity, and self-repression
- Scleranthus: inability to choose between alternatives
- Star of Bethlehem: shock
- Sweet Chestnut: extreme mental anguish, when everything has been tried and there is no light left
- Vervain: over-enthusiasm
- Vine: dominance and inflexibility
- Walnut: protection from change and unwanted influences
- Water Violet: pride and aloofness
- White Chestnut: unwanted thoughts and mental arguments
- Wild Oat: uncertainty over one's direction in life
- Wild Rose: drifting, resignation, apathy
- Willow: self-pity and resentment

Source: Adapted from: http://www.bachcentre.com/centre/remedies.htm, 2001.

Aromatherapy

Essential oils, comprised from plants (mostly herbs and flowers), can do wonders to relieve many hypothyroid symptoms naturally. The easiest way to use essential oils are in a warm bath; you simply drop a few drops of the oil into the bath, and sit and relax in it for about ten minutes. The oils can also be inhaled (put a few drops in a bowl of hot water, lean over the bowl with a towel over your head, and breathe); diffused (using a lamp ring or a ceramic diffuser—that thing that looks like a fondue pot); or sprayed into the air as a mist. You can use these oils for massage (you need a "carrier" base oil such as olive, jojoba, carrot-seed, grapeseed, or sweet-almond). You can also mix certain oils into a nonscented moisturizer and apply to your face (neroli, lavender, ylang-ylang, and rose all make for excellent "facial oils"). Twelve drops of oil in any of these methods is the average "dose." When oils are applied directly to the skin, two drops is the average. You can also rub the oils onto the soles of your feet (where the largest pores are), which will get them working fast!

The following essential oils are known to have calming, sedative, and/or antidepressant effects for hypothyroid-related depression: ylang ylang, neroli, jasmine, orange blossom, cedarwood, lavender (a few drops on your pillow will also help you sleep), chamomile, marjoram, geranium, patchouli, rose, sage, clary sage, and sandalwood.

The following scents are considered helpful in combating fatigue: clove, ravensara, rosemary, thyme, and basil.

The following scents are stimulating and energizing: lemon, grapefruit, peppermint, rosemary, and pine.

The following scents can improve circulation: birch, cinnamon bark, clary sage, cypress, hyssop, and nutmeg.

For intolerance to cold, try sandalwood in a bath.

To improve concentration, try basil, cedarwood, cypress, eucalyptus, juniper, lavender, lemon, myrrh, orange, peppermint, rosemary, sandalwood, or ylang-ylang.

For muscle aches, try birch, ginger, nutmeg, or rosemary.

To improve fingernails, try eucalyptus, grapefruit, lavender, lemon, melaleuca, myrrh, oregano, patchouli, peppermint, ravensara, rosemary, or thyme.

For sluggish digestion, rub a little fennel, nutmeg, sage, or tarragon on your stomach after eating.

For constipation try fennel, ginger, juniper, marjoram, orange, patchouli, rose, rosemary, sandalwood, tangerine, or tarragon.

To improve dry skin, try chamomile, geranium, jasmine, lavender, lemon, patchouli, rosewood, or sandalwood.

Take These to Heart

Hypothyroidism can cause high cholesterol, putting you at greater risk for cardiovascular problems. The following nutrients are good for strengthening or nourishing the heart.

- *Wheat germ oil.* One or more tablespoons/15 mL daily.
- *Vitamin E oil.* One or more tablespoons/15 mL daily.

- *Flaxseed (Linum usitatissimum)*, also known as linseed, is considered the best heart oil—but only if it is absolutely fresh and taken uncooked. One to 3 teaspoons/5 to 15 mL of flaxseed oil first thing in the morning is recommended. You can grind the seeds and sprinkle them on cereals or salads. You can also soak flaxseeds in water and drink the whole thing first thing in the morning.
- Other heart-protective oils can be found in the fresh-pressed oils of borage seed or black currant seed.
- Other essential fatty acids can be found in plantain, lamb's quarter, or amaranth.
- *Hawthorn berry tincture.* Take 25 to 40 drops of the berry tincture up to four times a day. Expect results no sooner than six to eight weeks.
- *Seaweed.*
- *Carotene-rich foods.* Look for bright-colored fruits and vegetables. The richer the color, the richer they are in carotene.
- *Garlic, knoblauch (Allium sativum).* The greatest heart benefits come from eating it raw, but you can also purchase deodorized caplets.
- *Lemon balm.* Steep a handful of fresh leaves in a glass of white wine for an hour or so and drink it with dinner. Or make lemon balm vinegar to use on your salads.
- *Dandelion root tincture.* Use 10 to 15 drops with meals.
- *Ginseng (Panax quinquefolium).* Chew on the root or use 5 to 40 drops of tincture.
- *Motherwort (Leonurus cardiaca).* Use a tincture of the flowering tops, 5 to 15 drops several times a day as needed.

Hands-On Healing

Improving your overall health goes a long way in managing hypothyroidism. You might consider adding a hands-on healer to your health care team. All ancient, non-Western cultures, be they in native North America, India, China, Japan, or ancient Greece, believed that there were two fundamental aspects to the human body. There was the physical shell (clinically called the corporeal body) that makes cells, blood, tissue, and so on, and then there was an energy flow that made the physical body come alive. This was known as the life force or life energy. In fact, it was so central to the view of human function that each non-Western culture has a word for "life force." In China, it is called qi (pronounced "chee"); in India it's called prana; in Japan it's called ki; while the ancient Greeks called it pneuma, which has become a prefix in medicine having to do with breath and lungs.

Today, Western medicine concentrates on the corporeal body and does not recognize that we have a life force. However, in non-Western, ancient healing, it is thought that the life force heals the corporeal body, not the other way around!

Just like the life force, every non-Western healer looks upon the parts of the body as "windows" or "maps" to the body's health. In China, the ears are a complex map, with each point on the ear representing a different organ and part of the psyche. In reflexology, the feet are "read" to tell us much about the rest of the body and spirit. In the Ayurveda, the tongue is read, while other traditions read the iris of the eyes, and so on. Western medicine doesn't really do this. Instead it looks at individual parts for symptoms of a disease and treats each part individually. So, let's say you notice blurred vision. You might go to an eye doctor and be given a prescription for glasses and sent on your way. But if this same person were to go to a Chinese medicine doctor, she would be told that the degeneration of her eyes points to an unhealthy liver. To the Chinese, the eyes are a direct window into the liver. (Interestingly, it is the eyes that turn yellow when you're jaundiced.) So, instead of a simple prescription for glasses, the Chinese healer will look into deeper causes of this liver imbalance in the body. You'll be asked about your personal relationships, your diet, your emotional well-being, and your job. And the treatment may involve a host of dietary changes, stress-relieving exercises, and/or herbal remedies. An Ayurvedic doctor may use the tongue to diagnosis the same liver imbalance, but the approach is the same. You'll be asked about your diet, lifestyle, work habits, and so on. In other words, the body is not seen as separate from the self. To a non-Western healer, what makes us who we are basically has to do with our individual personalities and our societal roles: Whom we marry, where we work, and how we feel about those things are just as important as our visual problems.

One of the most ancient forms of healing involves energy healing, which can include therapeutic or healing touch. Technically, these techniques are considered forms of biofield therapy. An energy healer will use his or her hands to help guide your life force energy. The hands may rest on the body, or just close to the body, not actually touching it. Energy healing is used to reduce pain and inflammation, improve sleep patterns and appetite, and reduce stress. Energy healing, supported by the American Holistic Nurses Association, has been incorporated into conventional nursing techniques with good results. Typically, the healer will move loosely cupped hands in a symmetric fashion on your body, sensing cold, heat, or vibration. The healer's hands are then placed over areas where the life force energy is unbalanced in order to restore and regulate the energy flow.

Therapies that help to move or stimulate the life force energy include:

- Healing touch
- Huna
- Mari-el
- Qi gong
- Reiki
- SHEN therapy
- Therapeutic touch

All forms of hands-on healing work in some way with the life force energy.

Massage

Massage therapy can be beneficial whether you're receiving the massage from your spouse or a massage therapist trained in any one of dozens of techniques, from shiatsu to Swedish massage. In the East, massage was extensively written about in *The Yellow Emperor's Classic of Internal Medicine*, published in 2700 B.C. (the text that frames the entire Chinese medicine tradition). In Chinese medicine, massage is recommended as a treatment for a variety of illnesses.

Swedish massage, the method Westerners are used to, was developed in the nineteenth century by a Swedish doctor and poet, Per Henrik, who borrowed techniques from ancient Egypt, China, and Rome.

It is out of shiatsu in the East and Swedish massage in the West that all the many forms of massage were developed. While the philosophies and styles differ in each tradition, the common element is the same: to mobilize the natural healing properties of the body, which will help it to maintain or restore optimal health. Shiatsu-inspired massage focuses on balancing the life-force energy.

Swedish-inspired massage works on more physiological principles: relaxing muscles to improve blood flow throughout connective tissues, which ultimately strengthens the cardiovascular system.

But no matter what kind of massage you have, there are numerous gliding and kneading techniques used along with deep circular movements and vibrations that relax muscles, improve circulation, and increase mobility. This is known to help relieve stress and often muscle and joint pain. In fact, a number of employers cover massage therapy on their insurance and health plans. Massage is becoming so popular, in fact, that the number of licensed massage therapists enrolled in the American Massage Therapy Association has grown from 1,200 in 1983 to more than 38,000 today. To find a licensed massage therapist, see the resources at the back of this book.

Massage is more technically referred to as soft-tissue manipulation. Some benefits of massage include:

- improved circulation
- improved lymphatic system
- faster recovery from musculoskeletal injuries
- soothed aches and pains
- reduced edema (water retention)
- reduced anxiety

Types of massage include:

- Deep-tissue massage
- Manual lymph drainage
- Neuromuscular massage
- Sports massage
- Swedish massage

Osteopathic Manipulation

Osteopathic manipulation is a hands-on healing technique utilized by an osteopathic practitioner. This involves many of the same kinds of hands-on diagnostic approaches used by a family doctor (pressing various points to gauge whether there's pain, difficulty breathing, and so on). But it also involves much more attention to things such as your posture and gait (the way you walk), overall flexibility and mobility, straightness of the spine, and so on. An osteopath will carefully examine your skin too, looking for fluid retention, muscular changes, temperature variations, and tenderness. The osteopath will then use hands-on healing techniques to manipulate and stimulate muscles, circulation, and so on. This may be combined with standard medical treatment in certain cases, but osteopathic manipulation tends to work well to relieve the physical symptoms of stress. One of the most common forms of osteopathic manipulation is "postural drainage," which is a technique used to mechanically unplug fluid blocks in the body to promote blood circulation.

Pressure Point Therapies

Pressure point therapies involve using the fingertips to apply pressure to pressure points on the body, believed to help reduce stress, pain, and other physical symptoms of stress or other ailments. There are different kinds of pressure point therapies; the most well known are acupuncture and reflexology.

Acupuncture is an ancient Chinese healing art that aims to restore the smooth flow of life energy (qi) in your body. Acupuncturists believe that your qi can be accessed from various points on your body, such as your ear, for example. Each point is also associated with a specific organ. Depending on your physical health, an acupuncturist will use a fine needle on a very specific point to restore qi to various organs. Each of the roughly two thousand points on your body has a specific therapeutic effect when stimulated. Acupuncture can relieve many of the physical symptoms and ailments caused by stress; it's now believed that acupuncture stimulates the release of endorphins, which is why it's effective at reducing stress, anxiety, pain, and so forth.

Western reflexology was developed by Dr. William Fitzgerald, an American ear, nose, and throat specialist, who talked about reflexology as "zone therapy." But in fact reflexology is practiced in several cultures, including Egypt, India, Africa, China, and Japan. In the same way as the ears are a map to the organs, with valuable pressure points that stimulate the life force, here the feet play the same role. By applying pressure to certain parts of the feet, hands, and even ears, reflexologists can ease pain, tension, and restore the body's life-force energy. Like most Eastern healing arts, reflexology aims to release the flow of energy throughout the body along its various pathways. When this energy is trapped, for some reason, illness can result. When the energy is released, the body can begin to heal itself.

A reflexologist views the foot as a microcosm of the entire body. Individual reference points or reflex areas on the foot correspond to all major organs, glands, and parts of the body. Applying pressure to a specific area of the foot stimulates the movement of energy to the corresponding body part.

Shiatsu massage also involves using pressure points. A healer using shiatsu will travel the length of each energy pathway (also called meridians), applying thumb pressure to successive points along the way. The aim is to stimulate acupressure points while giving you some of his/her own life energy. Barefoot shiatsu involves the healer using his foot instead of his hand to apply pressure. Jin shin jyutsu and jin shin do are other pressure point therapies similar to acupuncture.

You can work your own pressure points, too. Here are some simple pressure point exercises you can try.

• With the thumb of one hand, slowly work your way across the palm of the other hand, from the base of the baby finger to the base of the index finger. Then rub the center of your palm with your thumb. Push on this point. This will calm your nervous system. Repeat this using the other hand.

• To relieve a headache, grasp the flesh at the base of one thumb with the opposite index finger and thumb. Squeeze gently and massage the tissue in a circular motion. Then pinch each fingertip. Switch to the other hand.

• For general stress relief, find sore pressure points on your feet and ankles. Gently press your thumb into them, and work each sore point. The tender areas are signs of stress in particular parts of your body. By working them, you're relieving the stress and tension in various organs, glands, and tissues. You can also apply pressure with bunched and extended fingers, the knuckles, the heel of the hand, or a gripping motion.

• Use the above technique for self-massage on the hands, looking for tender points on the palms and wrists.

• Use the above technique to self-massage the ears. Feel for tender spots on the flesh of the ears and work them with vigorous massage. Within about four minutes the ears will get very hot.

Postural Reeducation Strategies

Another popular form of hands-on healing is using touch to guide your body into better posture and alignment, similar in some ways to chiropractic healing. Postural reeducation, as it is called, involves using touch. By learning better posture, coordination, and balance, structural and functional stress is relieved. Three of the most common postural reeducation methods used in North America are the Alexander technique, the Feldenkrais method, and Trager psychophysical integration.

The Alexander technique involves the repositioning of the head, neck, and shoulders. Developed by Shakespearean actor Frederick Matthias Alexander (1869–1955), it involves being verbally guided into better posture and alignment through exercises that may involve lying, sitting, standing, or walking. At the same time, you'll be given a hand on areas that have posture-related tension. By avoiding certain movements, you can greatly decrease back pain or back problems, improve overall health, and improve your mental health with better focus, more patience, and so on.

The Feldenkrais method was developed by physicist Moshe Feldenkrais. He believed that movement, thought, speech, and feelings are a reflection of self-image, and argued that people made aware of their habits related to motion can be taught to move more easily and gracefully, resulting in improved self-image and better health. A combination of verbal guidance and gentle touch are used to make you aware of customary movement patterns and possible alternatives. More graceful and aware movements can improve stress-related symptoms and overall health.

The Trager method was developed by Milton Trager, M.D. (1908–1997), and is often called the Trager Approach. This involves learning the joy of movement. Healers using this method use their hands to direct you through exercises involving bouncing, rocking, shaking, compression, and elongation. It is believed that using and moving your body in all the ways that it can be moved improves mindset, flexibility, overall health, and reduces stress-related tension. Trager was born with a congenital spinal deformity, and through this method he developed an athletic and graceful body.

Structural Integration

Developed by Ida Rolf, a biophysicist, Rolfing involves realigning bad posture caused by trauma or injury. A healer using the Rolfing technique will coax bones and muscles into proper alignment by using their thumbs, fingers, and elbows to deliver a sliding pressure to the affected area. Rolfing can cause some discomfort because it involves stretching the deep tissues sufficiently to bring the head, torso, pelvis, legs, and feet into alignment. But the results can be rewarding; stress can be greatly reduced or alleviated through Rolfing.

Where to Find (and How to Use) Hands-On Healers

If you're interested in trying one of these techniques, contact your family doctor or chiropractor for a referral. Naturopathic physicians are also a good source, and you can consult the resource list at the back of this book for specific organizations that can refer you to practitioners in your area. The "hairdresser" rules are also good ways of locating these practitioners; friends and family members who have had good experiences with any of these techniques are probably good resources.

When you find the practitioner in the discipline that interests you, be sure to tell the practitioner about any medications you're taking or other medical conditions. It's not recommended to seek out treatment while you have an active infection or virus such as a cold or flu. If you have inflamed or infected tissue, an infectious disease, a serious heart condition, or are undergoing treatment for cancer, consult your doctor before undergoing any of these therapies. *There is concern that some of these techniques could worsen some medical conditions.*

The benefits of many of these healing techniques are often not proven within standard Western studies. It's important to keep in mind that when it comes to researching alternative therapies, most Western researchers don't know enough about them to design proper studies. And many of these ancient disciplines just don't lend themselves well to Western-style research, such as double-blind controlled studies. There are other risks with alternative and complementary medicine that you should be aware of.

- There is no scientific proof to support most of the treatments you'll be offered, or claims of the therapies.

- Since there is no advisory board or set of guidelines that govern non-Western practitioners, the alternative "industry" attracts quacks and charlatans; as well, there can be prohibitive costs for some therapies.

- Academic credentials are all over the map in this industry. Beware of humbugs.

Self-Care

Dealing with hypothyroidism, or any disease, is stressful, which leaves us wide open to a number of ailments because of its effect on the immune system.

For example, we can suffer from stress-related

- allergies and asthma
- back pain
- cardiovascular problems
- dental and periodontal problems
- depression
- emotional outbursts (rage, anger, crying, irritation—seen in recent reports on "air rage" and "desk rage")
- fatigue
- gastrointestinal problems (digestive disorders, bowel problems, and so on)
- headaches
- herpes recurrences (especially in women)
- high blood pressure
- high cholesterol
- immune-suppression (predisposing us to viruses, such as colds and flu; infections; autoimmune disorders; and cancer)
- insomnia
- loss of appetite and weight loss
- muscular aches and pains
- premature aging
- sexual problems
- skin problems and rashes

As you can see from this lengthy list (in alphabetical order), stress can badly aggravate the already long list of hypothyroid symptoms (see Chapter 1). This section shows you ways to care for yourself during a bout of hypothyroidism, or anytime!

Eliminate Energy Drains

When you're hypothyroid, and dragging yourself around town, you need more energy rather than less. Among the worst "energy drains" are people. When you're surrounded by people who take energy from you, rather than give you energy in the form of support, the result is more stress in your life. By doing a serious reevaluation of your personal relationships, you may be able find more energy and reduce the amount of stress in your life. Ask yourself some of the following questions:

• Do you have someone in your life who offers judgment-free emotional support? This means a person who makes you feel positive about yourself rather than a person who points out your flaws or attacks your choices.

• Are there people in your life who drain your energy and reserves? These are people who always seem to be in crisis, and suck up large amounts of "free therapy" time from you, but never seem to be there for you. These can also be people who criticize you and make you feel negative and hopeless instead of positive and optimistic.

• Do you have unresolved conflicts with family members or friends? These unresolved feelings can drain your energy and focus as we tend to obsess about the conflict over and over.

• Is there a phone call you need to make, but are avoiding, that is causing you stress and anxiety?

• Is there someone in your life who continuously breaks commitments or plans, with whom you are constantly rescheduling?

Energy drains can also come from unmet needs in your home environment. Do you have broken appliances, car repairs that haven't been done, a wardrobe you hate, cluttered closets and rooms, or even ugly surroundings? Living in a home that is not decorated in a way that pleases you makes you feel as though you don't want to be there. Plants, paint, covers for ugly furniture, and a few things on the walls often make the difference between barren, dank surroundings and coziness.

Energy drains come from procrastinating and overbooking yourself. We will procrastinate over things we really don't want to do—such as taxes. We overbook ourselves when we're afraid of saying no. Every article and book on stress management has these three words of advice: "Just Say No." The problem is, few people will say it. Instead of no, try: "Let me check my schedule and see if I'm already committed." Then, "Sorry, looks like I'm committed elsewhere," or, if it's a task, "I've got a deadline on that date for something of equal importance."

Simply doing too much, and expecting too much from ourselves, drains our energy. When possible, hire someone to do the things you can't or don't want to do. When you're overworked at the office, subbing out one or two projects to a freelancer may be an ideal solution. If you don't think your employer will pay for the freelancer, have you considered subbing out the dreaded task on the sly, and paying for it out of your own pocket? The job security, perceived "good performance," and weight off your shoulders may be worth the cost. At home, have you considered hiring someone to:

- clean your house or apartment
- declutter your house by going through closets, filing things, and so on
- organize your tax receipts
- garden and/or take care of your lawn

Get Creative

Creativity can dramatically improve your sense of well-being. This refers to art in all its forms: words, fine arts, visual arts, healing arts, performing arts, hobbies, or sports. Writing, in particular, in the form of journal writing, poetry, or letterwriting is a stress-buster. A new study published in the *Journal of the American Medical Association* found that people suffering from chronic ailments such as asthma or arthritis actually felt better when they wrote about their ailments.

A few years ago, Oprah Winfrey used her influence to get her viewers to begin daily journal or diary writing because of the powerful way it can enable those of us who are otherwise without voice or expression. Using *her* own creativity to enable others, she has "resold" the idea of journaling in an age when few people take the time to sit down and be still with their thoughts. Oprah has taken it one step further by encouraging people to begin "gratitude journaling," where they think about what in their lives they are thankful for, and write it down. A firm believer in literacy as well, Oprah's influence on the comeback of journals can also enable many who in the past might have been afraid to write because of their education levels to find the courage to write and express themselves. For people who do not feel that they are "creative" or "artistic," journaling is an opportunity for anyone to express their feelings and passions.

Why is Martha Stewart so successful? Because she offers "creative rescue" for millions through her "lifestyle arts." She is essentially the "mountain" that comes to "Mohammed." Martha offers some "good things" that help change our days and routine. And when it's called *Martha Stewart Living*, there is the invitation to come back to life and feel the small things (which she'll tell you is a good thing), even if it's just to wake up and smell fresh coffee . . . *sorbet*. Whether it's beautiful flowers, crafts, or the hundreds of small things that take hours to make, she offers thousands of creative rescues every day through her program, magazine, and Web site.

Pamper Yourself

Taking care of yourself means being good to yourself. Give yourself some TLC. You'll find this goes a long way when you're hypothyroid. Here are some suggestions.

• Set aside "comfort time" for yourself at least once a week. Make it a ritual. It can be having coffee with your morning paper; going for a scenic stroll or "window shopping" in a favorite neighborhood; taking a long bath; going to an open market (these are often on the weekends); or having breakfast in bed once a week are all feel-good activities that will make you feel energized and loved.

• Have a very long shower some mornings. Treat yourself to a shower massage and take time to massage every part of your body. Buy energizing shower gels or shower "toys" to use.

• Have a steam bath. Run the shower and sit in your bathroom on a mat and just enjoy the steam.

• Have a luxurious bubble bath. Using aromatherapy to augment your bath can work wonders for relieving stress. For a spa-style bath, use mud products, dried milk powder for a milk bath, or mineral salts for aching muscles. The bath "ritual" can be enhanced with candlelight, and massaging oils or lotions to moisturize after the bath. Take a bed-rest day. Change the linens, fluff up your pillows, prepare good reading material, and a tray of good food (see Chapter 4). Spend the day as a "sick day" and rejuvenate.

- Plan a spa day (take this as a sick day if you like). Start your day in the bath (see above). Then go outside for a nice long walk. Come back inside and take an invigorating shower, scrubbing your body with a loofah scrubber or rough washcloth. Then wash your hair and put on a deep conditioning treatment. Leave the shower, stay in the bathroom, and begin to smooth the calluses on your feet. Start another bath with essential oils. (See "Aromatherapy" earlier in the chapter.) Cleanse your face well and apply your favorite facial mask. Light candles and soak, while putting a cool washcloth over your eyes. Then get back into the shower, rinse off the mask, and remoisturize your body. Wrap yourself in a towel and take a nap. (You may want to arrange in advance for a massage therapist to visit you at this point!) After your nap, make a nice "smoothie" with your favorite fruits. And then order in from your favorite restaurant to top off the day. Go to bed early with a book or magazine and a bed tray of snacks or the leftovers!

Appendix
For More Information

Note: Some of the addresses and phone numbers below may have changed since this list was compiled.

General

American Foundation of Thyroid Patients
P.O. Box 820195
Houston, TX 77282-0195
281-496-4460
Fax: 281-496-0369
www.thyroidfoundation.org
E-mail: thyroid@flash.net

ThyCa, Inc. (The Thyroid Cancer Survivors' Association)
P.O. Box 1545
New York, NY 10159-1545
877-588-7904 (toll-free)
Fax: 503-905-9725
www.thyca.org
E-mail: thyca@thyca.org
For membership information, E-mail membership@thyca.org.

Thyroid Foundation of America, Inc.
40 Parkman Street
Boston, MA 02114-2698
1-888-996-4460
www.tfaweb.org/pub/tfa
E-mail: tfa@clark.net

Thyroid Foundation of Canada
1040 Gardiners Road, Suite C
Kingston, Ontario
Canada K7P 1R7
1-800-267-8822
http://hom.ican.net/~thyroid/canada.html
E-mail: thyroid@limestone.kosone.com

Thyroid Society for Education and Research
7515 South Main Street, Suite 545
Houston, TX 77030
1-800-THYROID
www.the-thyroid-society.org
E-mail: help@the-thyroid-society.org

Autoimmune Disorders

American Autoimmune Related Diseases Association, Inc.
Michigan National Bank Building
14475 Gratiot Avenue
Detroit, MI 48205
313-371-8600
Fax: 313-372-1512

National Organization for Rare Disorders (NORD)
P.O. Box 8923
New Fairfield, CT 06812-1783
1-800-999-NORD
www.rarediseases.org

Congenital Hypothyroidism

CHAPS (Congenital Hypothyroidism and Parents' Support Group)
8 Rockhill Court
Edwardsville, IL 62025
618-692-1761

Graves' Disease

National Graves' Disease Foundation
2 Tsitsi Court
Brevard, NC 28712
704-877-5251, or send SASE with your information request
www.ngdf.org
E-mail: ngdf@citcom.net

Nederlandse Vereniging van Graves Patenten
Heemskerk Klein Elsbroek 3
2182 TE Hillegom
Holland

Hair Loss

American Hair Loss Council
1-800-274-8717

Buyer's Guide to Wigs and Hairpieces
c/o Ruth L. Weintraub
420 Madison Avenue, Suite 406
New York, NY 10017
212-838-1333

Edith Imre Foundation for Loss of Hair
30 West 57th Street
New York, NY 10019
212-757-8160

Wig Hotline
212-765-8397

Iodine Deficiency Disorders (IDD)

International Council for Control of Iodine Deficiency
   Disorders (ICCIDD)
J. T. Dunn, M.D.
Box 511, University of Virginia Medical Center
Charlottesville, VA 22908

Nuclear Medicine

Society of Nuclear Medicine
475 Park Avenue South
New York, NY 10016
212-889-0717

Thyroid Eye Disease

T.E.D. (Thyroid Eye Disease), Lea House
21 Troarn Way
CHUDLEIGH
Devon, UK TQ13 OPP
Phone/fax: 44-1626-852980
http://home.ican.net/~thyroid/international/TED.html

Thyroid Specialists

American Association of Clinical Endocrinologists
2589 Park Street
Jacksonville, FL 32204-4554
904-384-9490
Fax: 904-384-8124

American Thyroid Association, Inc.
Montefiore Medical Center
111 East 210th Street
Bronx, NY 10467
718-882-6047
Fax: 718-882-6085
Physician referral: 1-800-542-6687

The Endocrine Society
4350 East West Highway, Suite 500
Bethesda, MD 20814-4410
301-941-0200
Fax: 301-941-0259

Thyroid Federation International

Associazione Italiana Basedowiani e Tiroidei (Italy)
Australian Thyroid Foundation
National Graves' Disease Foundation (USA)
Schilddrusen Liga (Germany)
SCHILDKLIERSTICHTING Nederland (Netherlands)
Thyreoidea Landsforeningen (Denmark)
Thyroid Eye Disease Association (England)
Thyroid Foundation of America, Inc. (USA)
Thyroid Foundation of Canada
Vastsvenska Patientforeningen for Skoldkortelsjoka (Sweden)

Body Work/Hands-On Healing

American Academy of Medical Acupuncture
5820 Wilshire Boulevard, Suite 500
Los Angeles, CA 90036
1-800-521-2262
www.medicalacupuncture.org

American Academy of Osteopathy
3500 DePauw Boulevard, Suite 1080
Indianapolis, IN 46268-1136
317-879-1881

American Academy of Reflexology
606 East Magnolia Boulevard, Suite B
Burbank, CA 91501-2618
818-841-7741

American Chiropractic Association
1701 Clarendon Boulevard
Arlington, VA 22209
703-276-8800

American Massage Therapy Association
820 Davis Street, Suite 100
Evanston, IL 60201-4444
847-864-0123
Fax: 847-864-1178
www.amtamassage.org
E-mail: infor@inet.amtamassage.org

American Osteopathic Association
142 East Ontario Street
Chicago, IL 60611
1-800-621-1773; 312-280-5800
www.am-osteo-assn.org

Association for Network Chiropractic
444 North Main Street
Longmont, CO 80501
303-678-8086

International Chiropractors Association
1110 North Glebe Road, Suite 1000
Arlington, VA 22201
703-528-5000
www.chiropractic.org
E-mail: chiro@erols.com

International Institute of Reflexology
Box 12462
St. Petersburg, FL 33733
813-343-4811
E-mail: ftreflex@concentric.net

Jin Shin Do Foundation for Bodymind Acupressure
1048G San Miguel Canyon Road
Watsonville, CA 95076
408-763-1551

Jin Shin Jyutsu, Inc.
8719 East San Alberto Drive
Scottsdale, AZ 85258
602-998-9331
Fax: 602-998-9335

National Center for Complementary and Alternative Medicine
National Institutes of Health
8630 Fenton Street, Suite 1130
Silver Spring, MD 20910
1-888-644-6226
www.nccam.nih.gov

National Certification Board of Therapeutic Massage and Bodywork
8201 Greensboro Drive, Suite 300
McLean, VA 22102
1-800-296-0664; 703-610-9015
Fax: 703-610-9005
www.ncbtmb.com

North American Society of Teachers of the Alexander Technique
3010 Hennepin Avenue South, Suite 10
Minneapolis, MN 55408
1-800-473-0620; 612-824-5066

Nurse Healers—Professional Associates, Inc.
175 Fifth Avenue, Suite 2755
New York, NY 10010
212-886-3776

Office of Alternative Medicine Clearinghouse
Box 8218
Silver Spring, MD 20907-8218
1-888-644-6226
www.altmed.od.nih.gov

For Information About Federally Sponsored Research in Manual Therapies

The Feldenkrais Guild
524 Ellsworth Street, Box 489
Albany, OR 97321-0143
1-800-775-2118; 541-926-0572
www.feldenkrais.com
E-mail: feldngld@peak.org

The New Center College for Wholistic Health Education &
  Research
6801 Jericho Turnpike
Syosset, NY 11791
1-800-922-7337; 516-364-5533
Fax: 516-364-0989
www.newcenter.edu
E-mail: newcenter@d.com

Rolf Institute of Structural Integration
205 Canyon Boulevard
Boulder, CO 80302
1-800-530-8875
www.rolf.org
E-mail: rolfinst@aol.com

TRAGER Institute
21 Locust Avenue
Mill Valley, CA 94941
415-388-2688
www.trager.com
E-mail: admin@trager.com

Links from sarahealth.com

For more information about disease prevention and wellness, visit me online at www.sarahealth.com, where you will find over three hundred links—including these thyroid links related to your good health and wellness.

- ThyCa (Thyroid Cancer Survivor's Association): network of programs linking survivors and health care professionals around the world.
  www.thyca.org/home.htm

- American Foundation of Thyroid Patients
  www.thyroidfoundation.org

- Thyroid Foundation of Canada
  http://home.ican.net/~thyroid/canada.html

- Thyroid Foundation of America, Inc.
  www.tfaweb.org/pub/tfa

- American Thyroid Association
  www.thyroid.org

- Thyroid Disease Information Source: dozens of articles on everything related to thyroid disease, including conventional treatment and alternative drugs and therapies.
  www.digitalnation.com/mshomon.thyroid

- Mary Shomon's Thyroid Web site
  www.thyroid-info.com

- Medullary Support Group
  www.onelist.com/subscribe/medullary

- Anaplastic Support Group
  www.onelist.com/subscribe/anaplastic

- Thyroid Disease, Conditions, and Treatment: over two
  hundred pages of text and illustrations written by doctors for
  patients.
  www.thyroid.net

- Santa Monica Thyroid Diagnostic Center: very comprehensive
  site with patient and physician information, facts about
  nuclear medicine, cytopathology, and ultrasound.
  www.thyroid.com

- National Graves' Disease Foundation
  www.ngdf.org

- The Endocrine Society
  www.endo-society.org

- American Academy of Ophthalmology
  www.eyenet.org

- Thyroid Federation International: thyroid disease in a global
  perspective.
  www.thyroid-fed.org

- International Thyroid Group Home Page: information and
  support for fellow sufferers.
  www.my4tune.v-net.com/itg.htm

- Iodine Deficiency Disorders (International Council for the Control of IDD-ICCIDD)
  www.tulane.edu/~icciddhome.htm

- Congenital Hypothyroidism for Parents
  http://198.187.0.42/phl/newborn/chip.html

- Thyroid Disease Message Board: where people with all sorts of thyroid conditions and other endocrine problems swap information.
  www.healthboards.com.thyroid-disorders

- Hashimoto's Thyroiditis (Abbott Diagnostics): learn about signs, effects, and treatment.
  www.abbottdiagnostics.com/medical_conditions/thyroid/disorders/hashimoto.htm

- Hyperthyroidism @ HealthAnswers.com
  www.healthanswers.com/database/ami/converted/000356.html

Bibliography

Allardice, Pamela. *Essential Oils: The Fragrant Art of Aromatherapy.* Vancouver: Raincoast Books, 1999.

American Dietetic Association and National Center for Nutrition and Dietetics (NCND). "10 Tips to Healthy Eating." (April 1994).

"Armour Thyroid—Company E-mail Contact for Information." Posted online to http://thyroid.miningco.com/librar . . . kly/aa120998.htm?pid=2750&cob=home (February 8, 1999).

Berndl, Leslie, RD, MSc. "Understanding Fat." *Diabetes Dialogue,* 42, no.1 (Spring 1995).

Bower, Peter J., et al. "Manual Therapy: Hands-On Healing." *Patient Care* 31, no. 20 (December 15, 1997): 69.

"British Researcher Indicates That High Normal-Range TSH Values May Be 'Significant Departure from Normal.'" Posted online to http://www.bmj.com/cgi/content/full/314/7088/1175 (April 19, 1997).

Bunevicius, Robertas, et al. "Effects of Thyroxine as Compared with Thyroxine plus Triiodothyronine in Patients with Hypothyroidism." *New England Journal of Medicine* 340, no. 6 (February 11, 1999): 424–29.

Cass, Hyla, M.D. *St. John's Wort: Nature's Blues Buster.* New York: Avery Publishing Group, 1999.

"Cholesterol and Thyroid Disease." *Thyroid Signpost* 1, no. 2 (May 1993).

Costin, Carolyn, M.A., M.Ed., M.F.C.C. *The Eating Disorder Sourcebook.* Los Angeles: Lowell House, 1996.

Dadd, Debra Lynn. *The Nontoxic Home and Office.* Los Angeles: Jeremy P. Tarcher, 1992.

Delange, F. "Iodine Deficiency Disorders and Their Prevention: A Worldwide Problem." Abstract from the 6th International Thyroid Symposium, Thyroid and Trace Elements, 1996.

"Depression and Thyroid Disease." *Thyroid Signpost* 1, no. 3 (June 1993).

Dickens, B. M. "The Doctrine of Informed Consent." In *Justice Beyond Orwell,* edited by R. S. Abella and M. L. Rothman, 243–63. Montreal: Yvon Blais, 1985.

Dong, B. J., et al. "Bioequivalence of Generic and Brand-Name Levothyroxine Products in the Treatment of Hypothyroidism." *Journal of the American Medical Association* 277, no. 15 (April 16, 1997): 1199–200.

Emanuel, Ezekiel J., and Linda L. Emanuel. "Four Models of the Physician–Patient Relationship." *Journal of the American Medical Association* 267, no. 16 (1992): 2221–26.

"Endocrinology and Thyroid Disorders." Retrieved online from http://www.endo-society.org/pubaffai/factshee/thyroid.html (February 2, 1999).

Engel, June V., Ph.D., "Beyond Vitamins: Phytochemicals to Help Fight Disease." *Health News* (University of Toronto) 14 (June 1996).

———. "Eating Fibre." *Diabetes Dialogue* 44, no. 1 (Spring 1997).

Enzo, Iammetteo. "The Alexander Technique: Improving the Balance." *Performing Arts and Entertainment in Canada* 30, no. 3 (Fall 1996): 37.

Etchells, E., et al. "Disclosure." *Canadian Medical Association Journal* 155 (1996): 387–91.

———. "Voluntariness." *Canadian Medical Association Journal* 155 (1996): 1083–86.

————. "Consent." *Canadian Medical Association Journal* 155 (1996):177–80.

Ferraro, Cathleen. "New Uses of Chemicals Linked to More Illness." Published online Scripps-McClatchy Western (December 10, 1997).

Fransen, Jenny, R.N., and I. Jon Russell, M.D., Ph.D. *The Fibromyalgia Help Book*. Smith House Press, 1996.

Fraser, Elizabeth, R.D., C.D.E., and Bill Clarke. "Loafing Around." *Diabetes Dialogue* 44, no. 1 (Spring 1997).

Gaitan, Eduardo, M.D., F.A.C.P. "Goiter." *The Bridge* 10, no. 3 (Fall 1995).

Ginsberg, Jody, M.D., F.R.C.P. "Wilson's Syndrome and T3." *Thyrobulletin* 15, no. 4 (January 1995).

"Hair Loss and Thyroid Disease." *Thyroid Signpost* 1, no. 1 (April 1993).

Harrison, Pam. "Rethinking Obesity." *Family Practice* (March 11, 1996).

Hart, Ian R., M.B., Ch.B. M.sc., F.R.C.P.C., F.A.C.P., F.R.C.P. (Glas). "Does Your Patient Have a Thyroid Problem?" *Medicine North America* (February 1996).

Havas, S., and J. M. Hershman. "Action of Lithium on the Thyroid." Abstract from the 6th International Thyroid Symposium, Thyroid and Trace Elements, 1996.

Hetzel, Basil S., M.D. "Iodine Deficiency and Excess: A World Problem." *Thyrobulletin* 16, no. 3 (Fall 1995).

"High-Carbohydrate Diet Not for Everyone." Reuters: 16 April 1997.

Higley, Connie, Alan Higley, and Pat Leatham. *Aromatherapy A–Z*. Carlsbad, Calif.: Hay House, 1998.

Ho, Marian, M.Sc., R.D. "Learning Your ABCs, Part Two." *Diabetes Dialogue* 43, no. 3 (Fall 1996).

Hunter, J. E., and T. H. Applewhite. "Reassessment of Trans-Fatty Acid Availability in the U.S. Diet." *American Journal of Clinical Nutrition* 54 (1991): 363–69.

Hurley, Jane, and Stephen Schmidt. "Going with the Grain." *Nutrition Action* (October 1994): 10–11.

International Food Information Council. "Antibiotics in Animals: An Interview with Stephen Sundlof, D.V.M., Ph.D." (1997).

————. "Uses and Nutritional Impact of Fat Reduction Ingredients." *IFIC Review* (October 1995).

————. "Putting Fun Back into Food." (1997).

————. "Q&A About Fatty Acids and Dietary Fats." (1997).

————. "Sorting Out the Facts About Fat." (1997).

————. "What You Should Know About Aspartame." (November 4, 1996).

————. "What You Should Know About Sugars." (May 1994).

"Iodine Deficiency on Rise in U.S." *Journal of Clinical Endocrinology and Metabolism* 88 (October 1998): 3401–8.

Joffe, Russell, M.D., and Anthony Levitt, M.D. *Conquering Depression.* Hamilton: Empowering Press, 1998.

Knoll Pharma Inc. "The Many Aspects of Subclinical Hypothyroidism." (1995).

————. "The Many Faces of Undiagnosed Hypothyroidism." (1995).

Lark, Susan M., M.D. *Chronic Fatigue and Tiredness.* Los Altos, Calif.: Westchester Publishing Co., 1993.

Levine, R. J. *Ethics and Regulation of Clinical Research.* New Haven, Conn.: Yale University Press, 1988.

Lichtenstein, A. H., et al. "Hydrogenation Impairs the Hypolipidemic Effect of Corn Oil in Humans." *Arteriosclerosis and Thrombosis* 13 (1993): 154–61.

Martino, E., et al. "Increased Susceptibility to Hypothyroidism In-Patients with Autoimmune Thyroid Disease Treated with Amiodarone." *Clinical Thyroidology* VIII, no. 1 (January–April 1995).

Mastroianni, Anna C., Ruth Faden, and Daniel Federman, eds., *Women and Health Research: Ethical and Legal Issues of Including Women in Clinical Studies.* Volume 1. Washington: National Academy Press, 1994.

Matoo, T. K. "Primary Hypothyroidism Ecodary to Nephrotic Syndrome in Infancy." *Clinical Thyroidology* VIII, no. 1 (January–April 1995).

Mitchell, Marvin L., M.D. "Congenital Hypothyroidism." *The Bridge* 10, no. 4 (Winter 1995).

Nelson, Philip K., M.D. "Defining Chronic Fatigue Syndrome." *The Manasota Palmetto* (Sarasota, Fla.) January 1995.

"Nutrition News." *Diabetes Dialogue* 44, no. 1 (Spring 1997).

Olveira, G., et al. "Altered Bioavailability Due to Changes in the Formulation of a Commercial Preparation of Levothyroxine in Patients with Differentiated Thyroid Carcinoma." *Clinical Endocrinology* 46 (June 1997): 707–11.

"Recap of First Thyroid Cancer Conference Online." Posted online to http://thyroid.miningco.com/library/weekly/aa110298.htm (February 8, 1999).

"Research Finds Most Patients Feel Better with Addition of T3, Not Levothyroxine (i.e., Synthroid) Alone!!!" Posted online to http://thyroid.miningco.com/library/weekly/aa021199.htm?pid= 2750&cob=home (February 11, 1999).

Rosenthal, M. S. *Managing Your Diabetes*. Canada: Macmillan, 1998.

———. *The Gastrointestinal Sourcebook*. Chicago: NTC/Contemporary, 1998.

———. *The Type 2 Diabetic Woman*. Chicago: NTC/Contemporary, 1999.

———. *The Pregnancy Sourcebook*. 3rd ed. Chicago: NTC/Contemporary, 1999.

———. *50 Ways to Prevent Colon Cancer*. Chicago: NTC/Contemporary, 2000.

———. *50 Ways Women Can Prevent Heart Disease*. Chicago: NTC/Contemporary, 2000.

———. *The Thyroid Sourcebook*. 4th ed. Chicago: NTC/Contemporary, 2000.

———. *Women of the '60s Turning 50*. Toronto: Prentice-Hall Canada, 2000.

———. *50 Ways to Manage Heartburn and Reflux*. Chicago: NTC/Contemporary, 2001.

———. *50 Ways to Manage Stress*. Chicago: NTC/Contemporary, 2001.

Rudd, Wm. Warren, M.D. *Advice from the Rudd Clinic: A Guide to Colorectal Health*. Toronto: Macmillan Canada, 1997.

Self-Care Archives. "A Field Guide to Stress: A Conversation with Kenneth R. Pelletier, Ph.D." (December 15, 1997).

Seto, Carol, R.D., C.D.E. "Nutrition Labeling—U.S. Style." *Diabetes Dialogue* 42, no. 1 (Spring 1995).

Shimer, Porter. *Keeping Fitness Simple: 500 Tips for Fitting Exercise into Your Life.* Pownal, Vt.: Storey Books, 1998.

Shomon, Mary J. *Living Well with Hypothyroidism.* New York: Avon Books, 2000.

Singer, Peter A., M.D. "Hashimoto's Thyroiditis." *Thyrobulletin* 16, no. 1 (Spring 1995).

"Some Reasons for the Rise in Work Stress." Retrieved online from http://www.convoke.com/markjr/streesb.html (February 12, 1999).

Surks, Martin I., M.D. *The Thyroid Book.* Yonkers, N.Y.: Consumer Reports Book, 1994.

"Synthroid Under Siege." Posted online to http://thyroid.miningco.com/library/weekly/aa022499.htm?pid=2750&cob=home (February 24, 1999).

"The Return of Sunny Spring Isn't the Cure for All Cases of Seasonal Depression. Sometimes It's the Cause." Published online by Deborah Franklin. *Health Magazine* (1996).

Thyroid Foundation of America, Inc. Commentary on "Effects of Thyroxine as Compared with Thyroxine plus Triiodothyronine in Patients with Hypothyroidism." Retrieved online from www.tsh.org (February 17, 2000).

Thyroid Society for Education and Research. "Autoimmune Thyroid Diseases." *Thyroid Signpost* 1, no. 5 (August 1993).

Thyroid Society for Education and Research. "What About Tests and Treatment?. (1992).

Toft, Anthony, M.D. "Thyroid Hormone Replacement—One Hormone or Two?" *New England Journal of Medicine* 340, no. 6 (February 11, 1999): editorial.

University of California. "Olestra: Yes or No?" Excerpted from The University of California at Berkeley Wellness Letter in *Diabetes Dialogue* 43, no. 3 (Fall 1996).

Varl, B., J. Drinovec, and M. Bagar-Posve. "Iodine Supply with Mineral Water." Abstract from the 6th International Thyroid Symposium, Thyroid and Trace Elements, 1996.

Veatch, R. M. "Abandoning Informed Consent." *HCR* 25, no. 2 (1995): 5–12.

Walfish, Paul, M.D. "Thyroid Disease During and After Pregnancy." *Thyrobulletin* 16, no. 3 (Autumn 1995).

Westcott, Patsy. *Thyroid Problems: A Practical Guide to Symptoms and Treatment.* London: Thorsons/HarperCollins, 1995.

Willett, W. C., et al. "Intake of Trans-Fatty Acids and Risk of Coronary Heart Disease Among Women." *Lancet* 341 (1993): 581–85.

Wood, Lawrence C., M.D., David S. Cooper M.D., and E. Chester Ridgway, M.D. *Your Thyroid: A Home Reference.* 3d ed. New York: Ballantine Books, 1995.

Zellerbach, Merla. *The Allergy Sourcebook.* Los Angeles: Lowell House, 1995.

Index

147